The Black Death in England

The Black Death in England

Journal of the Plague Years in the Fourteenth Century

Kathryn Warner

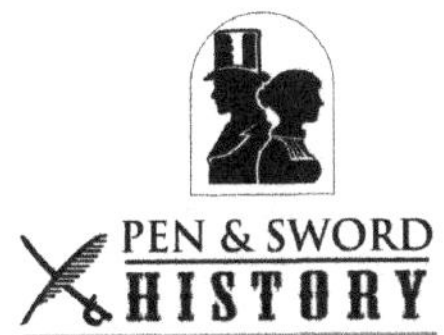

First published in Great Britain in 2025 by
Pen & Sword History
An imprint of Pen & Sword Books Limited
Yorkshire – Philadelphia

ISBN 978 1 03610 492 4

A CIP catalogue record for this book is available from the British Library.

Typeset by Mac Style
Printed in the UK by CPI Group (UK) Ltd, Croydon, CR0 4YY.

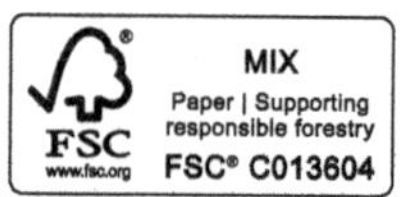

The Publisher's authorised representative in the EU for product safety is Authorised Rep Compliance Ltd., Ground Floor, 71 Lower Baggot Street, Dublin D02 P593, Ireland.
www.arccompliance.com

For a complete list of Pen & Sword titles please contact

PEN & SWORD BOOKS LIMITED
47 Church Street, Barnsley, South Yorkshire, S70 2AS, England
E-mail: enquiries@pen-and-sword.co.uk
Website: www.pen-and-sword.co.uk
or
PEN AND SWORD BOOKS
1950 Lawrence Road, Havertown, PA 19083, USA
E-mail: uspen-and-sword@casematepublishers.com
Website: www.penandswordbooks.com

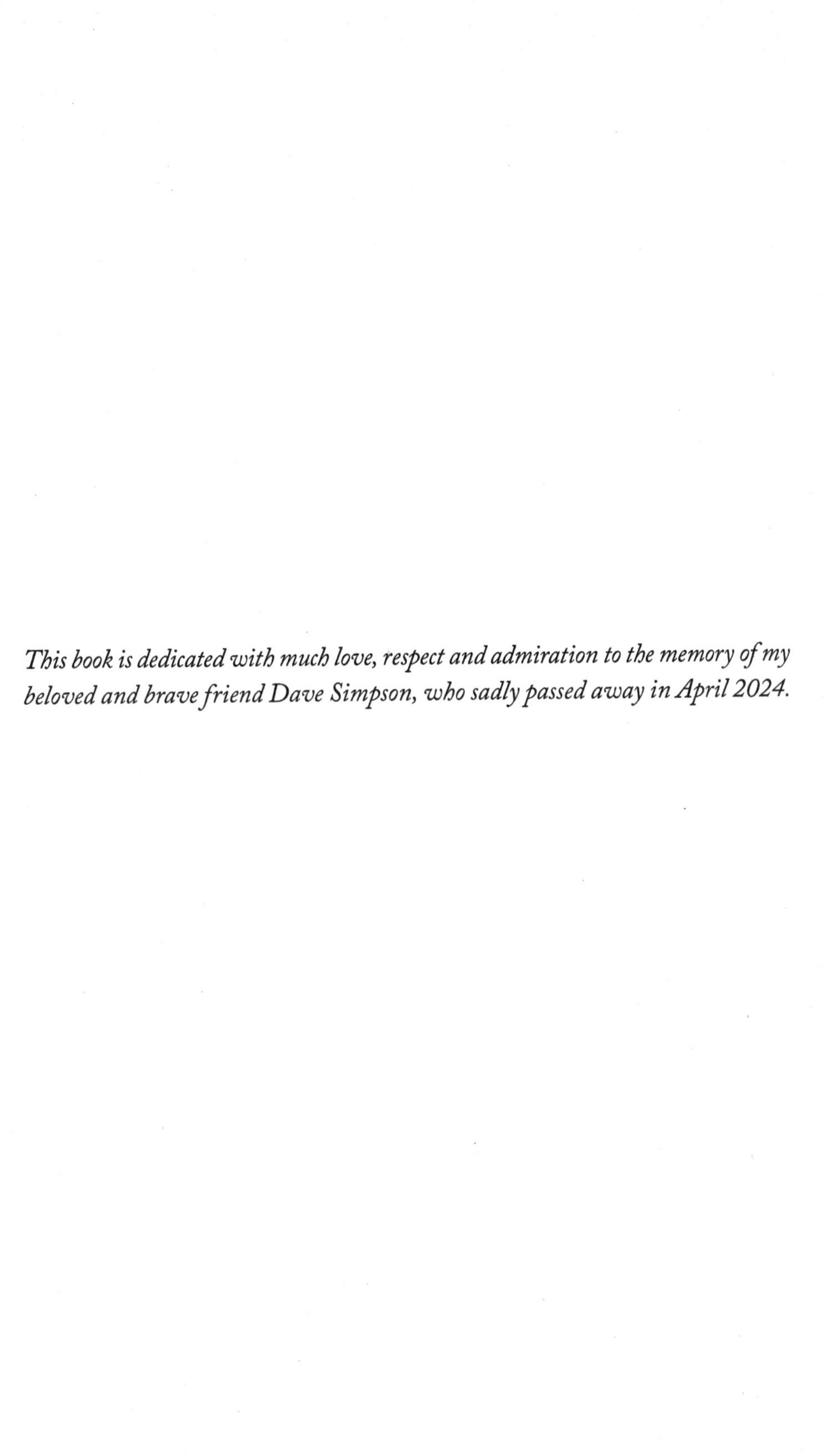

This book is dedicated with much love, respect and admiration to the memory of my beloved and brave friend Dave Simpson, who sadly passed away in April 2024.

Contents

Introduction

At the beginning of 1349, the Stokwell family lived on Whitecross Street (then called 'Whitecrouchestrete') in the parish of St Giles Cripplegate in London, a street that is now in the EC1 postcode and a few minutes' walk from the Barbican Centre. The family consisted of Walter, the father, Joan, the mother, Laurence, the only son, and four daughters, Christine, Imania, Alice and Agnes. Walter's brother William and sister Isabel were unmarried – or perhaps widowed – with no children, and both were close to Walter and his family. Walter Stokwell worked as a painter, or *peyntour* as it was spelt in his will, and instructed an apprentice, Thomas Bournham, who also lived in the household. Walter achieved success in his career, and he and his family were well-to-do. In his will, Walter bequeathed £5 (roughly £10,000 in modern terms) to his local church for a rich altar-cloth and £4 for another cloth to be used during funerals, arranged for sixty gold coins to be given to a person who wished to travel to the Holy Land on pilgrimage, gave a warm furred surcoat to his apprentice Thomas and dispensed alms to 'every religious order in the city of London', two hospitals and the paupers incarcerated in Newgate prison. The Stokwells led comfortable, even rather privileged, lives in the London of the mid-fourteenth century.

By the end of 1349, of the nine members of this happy, thriving family, only Agnes was still alive. She had lost her parents Walter and Joan, her brother Laurence, her older sisters Christine, Imania and Alice, her aunt Isabel and her uncle William; in short, every living relative. Agnes Stokwell was 7 years old.[1]

The endless tragedies of the Black Death are horrifying and unimaginable. The two sisters from Somerset, aged 12 and 13, who died hours apart on the same day. The grandmother, mother, stepfather and four daughters in Worcestershire who all died in the spring and early summer of 1349. The 6-year-old boy on the Isle of Wight who survived the first pandemic of 1348/49 that took his father, grandmother, step-grandfather and step-grandfather's son, only to die in another plague pandemic twenty years later. The family from Kent who all died within a few weeks in May and June 1349: both parents and all four of their daughters, the eldest of whom was just 5 years old. Suddenly a whole family was gone, wiped out by a terrifying disease.

One contemporary English chronicler called the Black Death 'a great mortality of men' (*magna mortalitas hominum*).[2] English records of the fourteenth century usually refer to it either as *mortalitas* or *pestilencia*, i.e., 'mortality' and 'pestilence', and the name 'Black Death' was not used in England for the disease until centuries later. Modern estimates of the number of victims in England during the first pandemic of 1348/49 vary wildly, though the most widely accepted figure for Europe in general is around 33%. In some places, however, such as eastern England, between 40% and 60% of the entire population perished in 1349.[3] The first pandemic of the Black Death in 1348/49 was by far the worst, though there were later outbreaks in England in the early 1360s, the late 1360s and the mid-1370s.

The Black Death in England: Journal of the Plague Years in the Fourteenth Century is not intended to be an account of the path the plague took through England and elsewhere, which has been brilliantly reconstructed and narrated in other books; see for example John Kelly's *The Great Mortality* and Benedict Gummer's *The Scourging Angel.* Nor does it provide an overarching view of what the pope said and did, what various English bishops said in 1349 or what chroniclers said, which amounts in most cases to declarations of how awful the plague was and how it killed numerous people, with few real details. This kind of information is easily found elsewhere, including on Wikipedia. Rosemary Horrox's *The Black Death* usefully provides translated primary sources from England and elsewhere, and articles on the Black Death appear regularly in the media and online. Nor is *Journal of the Plague Years* intended to be an account of the disease itself, i.e., the nature of the virus and how it spread, whether it truly was bubonic plague spread by rat fleas as has long been believed or something else like anthrax or an Ebola-like disease. S.K. Cohn's *The Black Death Transformed*, Barney Sloane's *The Black Death in London* and Gummer's *The Scourging Angel* are some of the works that discuss this important matter.[4]

It is very difficult to tell the social history of the Black Death in England, as so few sources exist. We have no diaries, very few letters and only a handful of narrative accounts written by chroniclers, which provide few if any details about the victims and their identities. Written records in England, did, however, continue to be kept through the plague years, at least in some places and in some circumstances, and though they are often chaotic, it is possible to piece different bits together and to tell the stories of some of the people who died as well as those who survived.

One important issue is that some forms of evidence simply do not exist from the fourteenth century. It is almost impossible to know how English people felt about the Black Death, whether they railed against their likely fate or fatalistically accepted it; whether or to what extent they turned to religion for comfort, or perhaps, in some cases, turned away from it; whether they realised that the plague was on its way to their village or town and tried to avoid it by fleeing, or instead decided that their best option was to hunker down in their homes and try to avoid everyone. In the fourteenth century, it is almost always the case that we do not know how people felt about anything, as most people were illiterate and had no means of recording their feelings, their fears, their hopes, their experiences. Of the many wills made in 1349, hardly any mention the plague directly, and the well-known English writers who lived through it, though it certainly altered their lives forever, almost never made a direct reference to it either. It must be realised, therefore, that English people's thoughts and feelings about their experiences during the Black Death are, in almost all cases, lost to us.

There are numerous examples of contemporary records that state that 'most of the inhabitants died in the pestilence' but without providing names of who these people were. Many modern books inform us that 'half the population of such and such town died', but with few if any names of the people who suffered and died in their thousands, it becomes difficult to feel much emotional connection to the numerous victims. They become mere statistics that blur into a kind of unreality, mute testimony to a catastrophe beyond imagination or comprehension. *Journal of the Plague Years* aims to give names to some of the people of England who died in the Black Death and those who lived through it, and to recreate a little of their lives wherever possible.

Part I

The Pandemic of 1348/49

Chapter 1

Before the Pestilence

The summer of 1348 was an extremely wet and chilly one in England, following a very wet winter and preceding another very wet autumn and winter. A chronicler named Ranulph Higden, based in Chester, stated that 'scarcely a day passed without it raining during the day or night' between the Nativity of St John the Baptist, i.e., 24 June, and Christmas that year.[1] Thomas Walsingham, a monk of St Albans, also wrote that 'there was a great downpour which lasted from Midsummer to Christmas' in 1348.[2]

King Edward III, born in November 1312, was 35 years old in that gloomy summer of 1348 and in the twenty-second year of his reign. A keen jouster, Edward held a tournament at Windsor Castle, his birthplace, in the last week of June 1348. His wife and queen, Philippa of Hainault, had recently borne their eleventh child, William of Windsor, and her purification or churching – a ceremony held about thirty or forty days after a woman gave birth – took place at Windsor Castle on 24 June. During the ceremony, Philippa wore a mantle, cape, supertunic and tunic of red velvet lined with costly ermine and miniver fur, while three of her sons, present at Windsor for her purification and their father's jousting tournament, also wore velvet garments.[3] This is an indication that June 1348 was an unusually chilly month; velvet and fur would normally have been far too hot at that time of year. Despite the awful weather, the Windsor jousts were a great success, and were attended by Edward III's brother-in-law David II, king of Scotland, a captive in England since his defeat at the battle of Neville's Cross in October 1346.

Fourteen-year-old Joan of Woodstock, the third eldest child of the English royal couple, was not present at the Windsor jousts, as she had set off for her wedding in Spain a few weeks previously. She was to marry Infante don Pedro, the 13-year-old heir to his father Alfonso XI's kingdom of Castile-León, and in late June 1348 was breaking her journey in Bordeaux, a city ruled by her father as duke of Aquitaine and later by her eldest brother the prince of Wales. The prince had given her three tuns of red wine for the journey as well as a brooch studded with rubies, diamonds, emeralds and pearls as a wedding gift, and during her journey south, Joan was accompanied by 130 archers from the West Country and a Spanish minstrel called Garcias Gyvill.[4] Among Joan's many siblings were Mary of Waltham, aged 3 years and 8 months in June 1348, and Margaret of Windsor, aged not quite 2, who were the youngest royal children other than the baby William of Windsor. All three of these royal daughters were destined to die during outbreaks of the Black Death.

England was officially at war with France in 1348. King Edward had claimed the French throne in 1337, and thus began what we know as the Hundred Years' War, and defeated Philip VI of France at the battle of Crécy in August 1346 (a few weeks before an English army led by Lord Neville and Lord Percy defeated David II of Scotland at Neville's Cross). In September 1347, following a long siege, Edward captured the port of Calais, which was to remain in English hands for the next 211 years. He arranged a truce with King Philip, which expired on 24 June 1348, the day of Queen Philippa's purification and the start of the jousting tournament at Windsor. As the truce was now no longer in force, Edward ordered all the sheriffs in England on 14 July to proclaim that 'no one shall tourney, joust or seek adventures or do other deeds of arms on pain of imprisonment', but should instead arm themselves and prepare to defend the realm against the French if necessary. Another, very short, truce was established between 13 September and 25 October 1348.[5]

In the mid-fourteenth century, England had a population of somewhere between 4.5 and 6 million inhabitants.[6] It was a long way from being a cultural wasteland, a barbaric ignorant backwater. A bright little boy named Geoffrey, who was about 5 or 6 years old in 1348, lived on Thames Street in London with his parents John and Agnes. Geoffrey's other relatives in London, people he would have known well, included his uncle Thomas Heyron, who was his father's older half-brother; his mother's cousin Nicholas Copton; and his step-grandfather Richard, the third husband and widower of Geoffrey's paternal grandmother, Mary. Vintry ward, where Geoffrey grew up, was a bustling, cosmopolitan area where many immigrants had settled, and his father and uncle both worked as wine merchants there. Geoffrey would live until 1400, and would write great works of literature that are still widely read in the twenty-first century. His last name was Chaucer.

One hundred and thirty miles northwest of London, in the Malvern Hills in Worcestershire, a young man named William Langland, aka William Rokele, was in his late teens or early 20s in 1348. He was of higher rank than Geoffrey Chaucer: his father Eustace 'Stacy' Rokele was a landowner in Shipton-under-Wychwood and elsewhere in Oxfordshire, and his grandfather Peter Rokele had served as a royal justice in Lincolnshire, owned lands in several counties and was very well-off; an abbot acknowledged in 1325 that he owed Peter £200.[7] At the time, the typical annual wage for a working man was in the region of £2 or £3. Like Geoffrey Chaucer, William Langland's name is still widely known today thanks to the great allegorical poem he wrote, *Piers Plowman*, a significant early work in the Alliterative Revival of the fourteenth and fifteenth centuries. It is apparent that Chaucer read *Piers Plowman* and was influenced by it, and Langland has been called one of the 'supreme poets of the European [M]iddle [A]ges'.[8]

Other talented English writers were alive in 1348. One was the anonymous Gawain Poet, who came from Cheshire or Staffordshire and wrote the poems *Gawain and the Green Knight* and *Pearl*, which were also alliterative and allegorical and are equally as highly thought of, many centuries later, as *Piers Plowman* is. Another was the anonymous author of *Wynnere and Wastoure* (*Winner and Waster*), a poem written around 1352 in the north Midlands or Lancashire, and yet another was John Gower, who was about 18 in 1348 and probably came from Kent or Suffolk. Unlike his contemporaries Chaucer, Langland, the Gawain Poet and the author of *Wynnere and Wastoure*, who wrote exclusively in English, the trilingual Gower composed his works in English, French and Latin. His best-known poem is the 30,000-line *Confessio Amantis*, A Lover's Confession, which was, despite its Latin title, written in English. Other English people of the era were also able to compose poems in Latin, including one whose modern title is 'An Invective Against France'. It was written in the aftermath of Edward III's victory over Philip VI at Crécy in 1346, with the aim of promoting the English king's claim to the French throne.

At Oxford University in the late 1340s, John Wycliffe, who was in his early 20s and had grown up in Yorkshire, was studying at Merton College. Merton was a centre of advanced mathematical and logical thought in the 1330s and 1340s, dominated by a group of men known to posterity as the Oxford Calculators. They included William Heytesbury from Wiltshire

(d. 1372/73), a Doctor of Theology who wrote the *Regulae solvendi sophismata* (*Rules for Solving Sophisms*); Richard Swineshead from Lincolnshire (d. *c.* 1354), who wrote the *Liber calculationum* (*Book of Calculations*) and inspired the German polymath Gottfried Leibniz more than 300 years later; Thomas Bradwardine from Sussex, who held four degrees, wrote numerous works on theology, geometry, arithmetic and motion, and briefly served as archbishop of Canterbury in 1349 before falling victim to the Black Death; and John Dumbleton from Gloucestershire, who wrote the *Summary of Logic and Natural Philosophy* and probably also died of plague in 1349.[9] John Wycliffe (d. 1384) also became a Doctor of Theology and is well-known for the unconventional religious beliefs he held and promoted, and for supporting the translation of parts of the Bible into Middle English. Later in the fourteenth century, John's followers the Lollards would be persecuted and, in the fifteenth, some of them were burned alive for heresy. One of the texts that John studied at Oxford was the *Summa logicae* (*The Sum of Logic*), which was taught to him by men who had themselves studied under its author, William Ockham or Occam, in the 1320s. William was a Franciscan friar from Surrey after whom Occam's Razor is named, and died in April 1347, the year before the Black Death reached England, aged about 60. William also held unconventional religious beliefs and, after John XXII excommunicated him, he spent the last few years of his life in Munich with the German emperor Ludwig of Bavaria, Pope John's most implacable enemy.

John Trevisa, a child growing up in Cornwall who was the same age as Geoffrey Chaucer, would attend Exeter College (founded 1314) at Oxford in the 1360s and would subsequently be employed as a vicar by Lord Berkeley of Berkeley Castle in Gloucestershire. A gifted translator, in the 1380s Trevisa would translate the *Polychronicon* of Ranulph Higden – who talked about the rainy weather in 1348 – from Latin into English, and was also an accomplished writer of original prose. Trevisa also made translations of scripture, which are considered forerunners to William Tyndale's sixteenth-century English Bible.[10] Walter Hilton, born around 1340/43, almost certainly studied at the University of Cambridge, and became an Augustinian canon at the priory of Thurgarton in Nottinghamshire. Hilton was a spiritual writer whose best-known work is *The Scale of Perfection*, and died in 1396.[11]

Julian (or Juliane or Juliana) of Norwich was the same age as Chaucer, Trevisa and Hilton, and also about 6 years old in 1348. She became an anchorite – a person who withdrew from the secular world to live a solitary and intensely religious, prayerful life – and wrote a book of devotions called *Revelations of Divine Love*, the oldest work in the English language known for certain to have been written by a woman. Towards the end of her life Julian was visited by the best known of the medieval English mystics, Margery Kempe, thirty years her junior, whose *Book of Margery Kempe* is considered the first autobiography in English. Julian was surely aware of two other mystics and religious writers from Yorkshire who were a few years older than she: Richard Rolle, a hermit who was born *c.* 1300/1310 and died in September 1349 during the Black Death, and Richard's chief follower Margaret Kirkby, an anchorite who promoted Richard's unofficial cult in Yorkshire after he died. Richard Rolle left the University of Oxford without graduating after a religious conversion and returned to his native Yorkshire, where he made himself a habit out of his sister's gowns and preached in the town of Pickering, then became a religious recluse. Like his younger contemporaries John Wycliffe and John Trevisa, Richard was deeply interested in translating scripture and translated the Psalms into Middle English, as well as composing original texts in both Latin and his native English. One of these was a guide for religious recluses addressed to Margaret Kirkby personally. Margaret, in her 20s when Richard died at the end of the 1340s, lived into the 1390s.[12]

Alongside the many talented poets, translators and mathematicians, and those whose writing helped to ignite the first tiny sparks of the English Reformation, gifted artists and sculptors were hard at work in the England of the mid-fourteenth century. Sir Geoffrey Luttrell of Lincolnshire, who died in 1345, commissioned the magnificent and lavishly illustrated piece of art known as the Luttrell Psalter, now in the British Library, which provides numerous fascinating insights into English rural life of the era. Other beautiful contemporary psalters still survive today, including two that belonged to Edward III's mother Isabella of France (d. 1358), and another known as the Tickhill Psalter. Many effigies made in the fourteenth century also still exist in the twenty-first. The tomb and effigy of Edward III's father Edward II in St Peter's Abbey, Gloucester (now Gloucester Cathedral), made in the 1340s, are among the greatest treasures from medieval England that we can still admire today. Another spectacular contemporary example is the effigy of Blanche Mortimer, Lady Grandison, which can be seen in the church of St Bartholomew in the village of Much Marcle, Herefordshire. Blanche died in her 20s or early 30s in 1347. Her effigy depicts a beautiful, serene young woman who clutches a rosary in her left hand and wears a cloak over a gown with tightly buttoned sleeves. Her hair, covered by a head-dress that frames her face, is in coiled bunches at each side of her head, as was the fashion at the time. Cleverly, the gifted sculptor made Blanche's gown look as though it is spilling over the side of the tomb-chest. A chronicler named John of Reading would have approved of the modest choice of clothing; describing the 1340s, he wrote that English men and women alike wore their clothes far too short and tight and that they copied the look of decadent foreigners, and women had to wear foxtails hanging under their skirts 'to hide their arses'.[13] The equally disapproving Henry Knighton, a chronicler from Leicester, claimed that several dozen highly born women caused heavy thunderstorms that disrupted Edward III's jousting tournaments, and were even responsible for the Black Death, because they dressed in 'amazing men's clothes'.[14]

A famous English physician named John Gaddesden, another graduate of Merton College at Oxford – in theology as well as in medicine – was in his late 60s in 1348. He wrote a medical compendium called the *Rosa Medicinae*, cured one of Edward I's sons of smallpox in the early 1300s and is believed to have been the model for Chaucer's 'doctour of phisik' in his *Canterbury Tales*. John lived through the first pandemic of the Black Death and died in 1361 when he was about 80. His book cites Galen extensively and contains few real medical insights, hardly surprising for the era in which he lived, given that the 1340s was a decade in which a coroner's report stated that one Henry Callere 'was going upstairs alone when he fell down and died' as though this was a sufficient explanation for a sudden and unexpected death.[15]

Contrary to the popular modern belief that everyone in the Middle Ages died relatively young, there were many other long-lived people in the fourteenth century besides John Gaddesden. Pope Clement VI stated in March 1348 that the dean of London, Gilbert Bruer, was '80 years old, and infirm'. Gilbert was still alive in July 1351. Hamo Hethe served as bishop of Rochester from 1319 until his resignation in 1352, in 1353 was said to be over 80 and was alive in May 1357.[16] Edward III's cousin Margaret de Bohun was born in 1311 and died in 1391, her husband Hugh Courtenay, earl of Devon, was born in 1303 and died in 1377 and another royal cousin,

Margaret of Norfolk, countess of Norfolk in her own right, was born in *c.* 1322 and died in 1399. The French noblewoman Marie de St Pol, countess of Pembroke, was an exact contemporary of Hugh Courtenay. She was born in 1303 or 1304, moved to England in 1321, was widowed in 1324, founded Pembroke College at the University of Cambridge in 1347 and died in 1377. Joan Lovell, née Ros, died on 13 October 1348 at what must have been an advanced age; she gave birth to her son, who was killed at the battle of Bannockburn in June 1314, in 1288. Joan outlived her grandson, born in *c.* September 1314 as her son's posthumous son, by almost a year, and her heir was her great-grandson John Lovell, 7 years old in 1348.[17] Simon Simeon, steward of the earls of Lancaster, was born before 1310 and died in 1386 or 1387; the thrice-married Margaret Hydon from Devon was born before 1278 and died in 1357, when her heirs were her 38-year-old grandson and her great-granddaughters; and William Causton, a merchant working in London, was old enough to have qualified as a master of his trade and to act as someone's executor in 1306, and lived until 1354. In fourteenth-century London, nobody over the age of 70 was allowed to serve on juries or assizes, a rule that would hardly have needed to exist if virtually nobody reached such an age.[18]

Edward III held two parliaments in 1348, both at Westminster – which was by no means a given in the fourteenth century, when parliament took place wherever the itinerant king happened to be at the time. The second of the year, held in April 1348, would be the last one for almost three years; the next parliament would take place in February 1351, after one summoned to be held in January 1349 was at first postponed several times then cancelled altogether because of the plague. One petition presented to parliament in 1348 complained that 'it is notoriously known throughout the counties of England that robbers, thieves and other criminals travel and ride on foot and horse ... and commit thefts and robberies'.[19] In March 1348 as a result of another petition presented to him in parliament, King Edward ordered an investigation into the obstruction of 'the four great rivers of England, Thames, Severn, Ouse and Trent' by numerous weirs, mills, 'piles and palings' and other building work, which prevented ships and boats passing.[20]

Also in March 1348, Edward ordered the sheriff of Middlesex to proclaim that 'all those who have the taint of leprosy' were to be banished from the roads and fields between London and Westminster. The two places were then two miles apart, and 'there is a continual passage of magnates, justices, clerks and other ministers of the king's court' between them, Edward wrote. The sheriff was to take a group of men 'who have most knowledge of this disease' and would identify those with leprosy, and transfer them to 'solitary country places', as their presence between London and Westminster caused 'manifest danger' to those passing. Two years earlier, the king had banished lepers from London, claiming that they actively endeavoured to contaminate others 'by the contagion of their polluted breath ... [and] by carnal intercourse with women in stews [brothels] and other secret places'.[21]

In Great Yarmouth (then called 'Jernemuth') on 22 April 1348, the day after Easter Monday, five commissioners found that although there had been ninety 'great ships' in the port twenty years earlier, there were now only twenty-four, plus a few 'old broken ships lying on the sand, which their owners cannot afford to repair'. The rest had either been commissioned by Edward III for his war against France and been sunk or badly damaged in action, or had been lost in storms; one of the ships lost was the *Godyer*, 'Goodyear', and another was the *Plentee*, 'Plenty'. As a result, 'several of those who live in the town and were formerly well-to-do scarcely have a living'. Some men had been forced to leave the town and seek their livelihood elsewhere, including Benedict Shepwryghte, Richard Walsham, Thomas Thurleton and John Parle. Another inquisition was held in the tiny Kent hamlet of *Shyngledewelle* or Singlewell south of Gravesend on 25 June 1348. The sheriff of Kent and three others found that, in August 1344, Sir Thomas Ovedale had stayed in his friend William Chapman's home in Singlewell, and that Thomas's careless servants started a fire that burned down William's house and those of his neighbours. One of the houses badly damaged by fire belonged to the local coroner, Michael Ifield, and a chest where Michael kept his documents, rolls and memoranda was destroyed. Happily, fourteenth-century England was a society that placed a high value on the written record, and all the coroners of Kent kept copies of each other's documents, so that nothing was permanently lost.[22]

The year 1348 was a normal year when English people were born, married and died, were the victims and perpetrators of crime, suffered accidents, squabbled with their neighbours, and so on. Ralph of Cambridge appeared before the Assize of Nuisance in London on 1 August 1348 and complained that the common wall between his home and his neighbour

William Brangweyn's was not thick enough. As a result, sewage from William's latrine 'penetrates and defiles his whole premises'. William was ordered to build a stone wall two and a half feet thick. A few weeks later, William Peverel of Candlewick Street in London told the Assize that his neighbour Maud atte Vine had built an extension on her house that blocked the light of his windows. Maud protested, hardly unreasonably, that she had extended her own house that stood on her own land, which she had every right to do, and thus had no case to answer.[23] The Assize of Nuisance in London was held on Fridays every few weeks by the mayor and some of the two dozen aldermen. The mayor of London in 1348 was Thomas Leggy, who served until 28 October 1348 when he was replaced by John Lovekyn in the annual mayoral election, which always took place on that date, the feast of St Simon and St Jude. Thomas's brother Peter Leggy was to die in 1349 during the Black Death. Thomas himself was a skinner by trade, i.e., a person who prepared and sold animal skins, was married twice to women called Margaret and Alice, and had two sons who confusingly were both named Simon. Another Simon, also a London skinner and an associate of Thomas Leggy, was Simon Pulham, who was alive in July 1346 and died before early December 1348, when his widow Katherine married her second husband, skinner Nicholas Bole. Katherine in turn was dead by March 1351 when Nicholas was married to a woman named Agnes.[24]

John Stratford, archbishop of Canterbury, died on 23 August 1348, one assumes of natural causes rather than the plague given that Stratford, another long-lived person of the era, was over 70 at the time of his death. John Ufford was elected the following month. King Edward's 18-year-old cousin John of Kent, earl of Kent, married the German teenager Elisabeth von Jülich, a niece both of Queen Philippa and the emperor Ludwig of Bavaria, in or shortly after April 1348. John died childless in 1352; Elisabeth, yet another person who lived a long life, did not die until 1411. In early 1349, Edward III appointed Elisabeth's father Wilhelm von Jülich to negotiate a marriage between his and Queen Philippa's eldest daughter Isabella of Woodstock (b. 1332) and the widowed Charles IV, king of Germany, Italy and Bohemia, who founded the Charles University in Prague in 1348. This did not work out; Charles married Anna of the Palatinate instead.[25] And Alice de Lacy, countess of Lincoln in her own right, passed away on 2 October 1348, aged almost 67.[26] Her eventful life included walking out on her royal first husband

Thomas of Lancaster – who was later beheaded by his cousin Edward II – making a love-match with her second husband, who was far beneath her in rank, and being abducted by her third and forcibly married to him.

Alice's large inheritance passed to her nephew-in-law Henry of Grosmont, earl of Lancaster, Leicester and Derby, who was in his late 30s and was the third member of the recently established Order of the Garter after Edward III and his eldest son the prince of Wales. In 1354, now the first duke of Lancaster, Henry would compose a remarkable treatise in French titled *The Book of Holy Medicines* (*Le Livre de Seyntz Medicines*). It reveals much about him as a person, including his love of wearing rich cloth, eating salmon, smelling roses, dancing, kissing women and stretching out his calves in his stirrups at jousting tournaments so that women would admire them, and his dislike of getting up early to hear Mass. Henry's daughter and ultimate heir Blanche of Lancaster, who was 6 in 1348 and would become the mother of King Henry IV nineteen years later, is memorialised in the *Book of the Duchess*, the first work written by her contemporary Geoffrey Chaucer. Blanche's aunt Eleanor of Lancaster, fifth of Henry of Grosmont's six sisters, married her second husband Richard Fitzalan, earl of Arundel, in 1345 and gave birth to five children between 1346 and 1353. Six hundred years later, Eleanor and Richard's effigies with joined hands in Chichester Cathedral inspired Philip Larkin's poem 'An Arundel Tomb'.

Pope Clement VI wrote to Henry of Grosmont on 14 July 1348 regarding Henry's household retainer Sir Robert Corbet. Henry had notified the pope that Robert had once been rich and powerful, but 'by reason of his great liberality when marrying his sons and daughters, is now come to want' and was 'labouring under perpetual infirmity' to boot. Robert wished his only unmarried daughter, Amice, 'elegant and fair', to wed one Edward Strange, but the couple were third cousins. Clement told Henry of Grosmont that he had issued a dispensation for consanguinity so that the couple might marry. A few months later in March 1349, Henry asked Clement to issue another dispensation for Elizabeth (b. October 1338), daughter and heir of Lord Segrave, to marry John (b. June 1340), son and heir of Lord Mowbray. The two lords were quarrelling, and the marriage of their children would, Henry claimed, help to bring about peace between them.[27] Elizabeth and John did marry, and their son Thomas Mowbray, duke of Norfolk, appears in the opening scenes of Shakespeare's play about Richard II, Edward III's grandson and successor.

Katherine Barker married John Conegreve in Penkridge, Staffordshire on Monday, 12 May 1348, Roger and Alice Newebrugge married also in Penkridge on 16 May, and Alice Lenard married William Cok in Chalfont St Giles, Buckinghamshire on Friday, 5 September. Thomas Trewyk was born in Kibblesworth, Northumberland on 24 November, John Cokheved was born in Barton-upon-Humber on 20 December, and Thomas in the Wylowes (Willows) died in Barrington, Cambridgeshire on 30 April, leaving his house and 30 acres of land to his 27-year-old son Thomas the younger. The inquisition post mortem of William atte Solere of East Grinstead in Surrey, who died on 3 December 1347, was belatedly held on 15 September 1348, and it was found that his infant daughter Alice, born in February 1347, was heir to his house and three meadows. Alyna, widow of William of Bolingbroke in Lincolnshire, died in early 1348, a year after her husband had passed away, leaving their daughters Sarra, Katherine, Juliana and Joan and their grandson William, Sarra's son. Shortly after her mother's death, Joan, the youngest daughter, married John Sporoun, an apprentice goldsmith. John of Croydon, a successful and extremely well-off fishmonger, died at the end of 1347, leaving behind a large family: wife Lucy, daughters Alice, Nicholaa, Margaret, Joan and Margery, sons William and John, granddaughter Lucy, son-in-law Geoffrey Horn and siblings Gunnora, Hugh and William. An inquisition held in Croydon on 21 February 1348 found that John's elder son William, born in February 1334, was heir to his 56 acres of land in Croydon and a house in Southwark, and John left £50 – something like £100,000 in modern terms – to each of his daughters. John's brother Hugh of Croydon, also a fishmonger, was to die at the height of the Black Death in the spring of 1349. Hugh and his wife Margery had a daughter, Juliana, and two sons, both named John; one was a fishmonger and the other a goldsmith.[28]

Richard Nicoles suffered a misfortune in 1348 when his house in Shareshill near Wolverhampton burned down, and Geoffrey Cokerel was attacked and robbed by thieves in the Essex village of Little Laver. Geoffrey may be the man of this name who was sentenced to death for larceny and hanged around this time, but when he was taken to the nearby churchyard for burial, 'he miraculously, as is said, revived'. Edward III pardoned him in April 1349. Juliana Fetherwif also obtained a royal pardon for stealing a horse worth

10 shillings and thus escaped execution, Thomas Swetcok drowned in a pond in Earls Barton in Northamptonshire, and not long before 10 April 1348 the unusually named Seman Stok was murdered in his home in Ashby St Ledgers, also in Northamptonshire: Henry Wycok shot him in the throat with an arrow and fled.[29]

In the Nottinghamshire village of Oxton, the equally unusually named Sampson Strelley turned 14 on 3 July 1348, had a son Nicholas in 1353 and lived until 11 February 1390. Nicholas Strelley, son of a teenage father who lived through the Black Death, died on 21 September 1430 at the age of 77. Nicholas Bokton, who had grown up in Sandwich in Kent and was at the start of his teens, moved to the small Hampshire village of Itchen Abbas near Winchester to begin an apprenticeship as a tailor in or not long before 1348. In Woodford in Northamptonshire, Alice and Thomas Boson had an infant son, Henry, whose first birthday fell on 30 September 1348, and Bartholomew atte Cros, who also lived in Woodford with his parents Richard and Alice, was just a few weeks younger than Henry Boson. Bartholomew would survive the first pandemic and take the habit of a monk at the Cistercian abbey of Pipewell in Northamptonshire in his teens in 1362. Another resident of Woodford was 22-year-old Richard Cotty, who was mourning his sister Alice Cotty. During the winter of 1347/48, she walked the three miles to the market in Thrapston and perished on her way home when caught in a sudden snowstorm. Her body was retrieved from under a pile of snow and examined by the coroner.

Thirty-one-year-old John Lavele of Ugley in Hertfordshire was also mourning: his wife Isabel 'lay down on her bed and died suddenly' while he was at church on Christmas night in 1347. Roger Sulbek of Messing in Essex, who was about 21, was recovering from a broken leg, having managed to fall into a pit on his way to church that same Christmas night. (Roger survived both the broken leg and the pestilence, and was still alive in the late 1360s.) Thomas and Isabel Daniel's daughter Margaret was born in Bradley, Cheshire on 9 June 1348, though the family soon moved to Aikton in Cumberland, eight miles from Carlisle. Both Thomas and Isabel died in Aikton in the autumn of 1349, almost certainly of the plague, leaving Margaret an orphan at less than 18 months old. Another Margaret, the daughter of Peter and Agatha Blount, turned 2 years old in Chilfrome, ten miles from Dorchester, on 29 July 1348. Her parents also seem to have died in the Black Death, her grandfather Thomas Blount died in early 1350, her older brother John died as a child in 1353 and she married Walter atte More when she was 14.

In Bolton-by-Bowland in the Ribble Valley (then in Yorkshire, now in Lancashire), two cousins, Margaret Fauvel and Ellis Fauvel, both turned a year old in November 1348. Margaret Strayte of Bamburgh in Northumberland died on 15 August when her son John was about 4, and Katherine Bakwell of Mottingham in Kent died on 9 December, also leaving a son named John, who was about 3 years old. Katherine's widower Thomas Bakwell married a second wife named Elizabeth and had two more sons, William and Robert, before he died in 1361. John Gylessone from Reepham in Norfolk was sentenced to be locked in the pillory for an hour in May 1348 for selling 'putrid and stinking meat' to Agnes Ismongere, i.e., Ironmonger in modern English. Revoltingly, he had come across a dead sow in a ditch, flayed it and sold its meat. During John's time in the pillory, what was left of the meat was burned beneath him, the customary punishment for those who sold rotten food to the public.[30]

This, then, was England in 1348: a land that produced great writers, artists, mathematicians and thinkers, a land whose armies had very recently defeated French and Scottish armies, and a land where the female half of the population could and often did inherit and own property. It was also a land where leprosy and smallpox existed, where thieves were hanged, and where people were sentenced to have rotten meat burned beneath them in public while their head and hands were locked into a wooden contraption. A land where people lived and loved, danced and sang and laughed, and which was shortly to experience the greatest pandemic in history. A dread disease was on its way to England.

Chapter 2

Arrival of the Pestilence

Precisely when and where the Black Death arrived in England in the summer of 1348 is difficult to say for certain. With the usual medieval habit of giving a date as an important Christian feast day rather than the calendar date, chroniclers say that the plague arrived on the Nativity of St John the Baptist, which is 24 June, the Translation of St Thomas Becket the Martyr, which is 7 July, or the feast of St Peter in Chains, which is 1 August. The port of Melcombe (now called Melcombe Regis and part of Weymouth) in Dorset is given by several chroniclers as the plague's entry point, while others say Bristol.[1] Both make sense; Bristol was a major port with numerous ships from all over Europe travelling and trading there, while Melcombe had strong links with Calais, the French port that Edward III had captured the previous year.

One of the earliest English plague victims was 14-year-old Joan of Woodstock, the king and queen's third eldest child and second daughter. She died in Bordeaux on or a little before 1 July 1348 of what chronicler Geoffrey le Baker calls the 'great pestilence', *magna pestilencia* in the Latin original (Baker also describes the 'small black pustules' (*pustulos parvos nigros*) that were seen all over the bodies of Black Death victims).[2] Joan never met her Spanish fiancé Infante Pedro, and never saw the land of which she should have become queen. Her grieving father King Edward sent moving letters expressing his grief to Pedro and his father King Alfonso on 15 September, and another to his mother Queen María on 12 October.[3] And King Edward and Queen Philippa were to experience more bereavement in 1348 when their infant son William of Windsor died too, perhaps on 9 July. His funeral took place at Westminster Abbey on 5 September.[4] Whether Joan of Woodstock would have had a happy marriage with Pedro of Castile-León is impossible to say, though it seems rather unlikely. Three years after he succeeded his father on the throne as a 15-year-old in March 1350, Pedro married the French noblewoman Blanche de Bourbon, but imprisoned her mere days after their wedding to go off with his mistress, doña María de Padilla, with whom he had four children. King Pedro and doña María's daughter Isabel moved to England in the early 1370s and became duchess of York by marriage to Joan of Woodstock's brother Edmund of Langley, and was a great-grandmother of the English kings Edward IV (r. 1461–83) and Richard III (r. 1483–85).

Hugh Courtenay, eldest child of the earl and countess of Devon and one of the founding members of the Order of the Garter, a kinsman of Joan of Woodstock, is another likely early victim of the plague. Hugh was born on 22 March 1327, twelve days before his mother Margaret de Bohun, a cousin of Edward III, turned 16. In the early 1340s, Hugh married Elizabeth, daughter of John de Vere, earl of Oxford (b. 1312), and their son was born around 1345. Hugh died sometime after Easter 1348 and before August 1349, aged 21 or 22, and was buried at Forde Abbey in Dorset. As the abbey lay only thirty miles from Melcombe, it is generally assumed that he died of the Black Death.[5] His long-lived parents did not die until 1377 and 1391, his widow Elizabeth married again twice before she died in 1375 and his son, who would have succeeded his grandfather as earl of Devon if he had lived three years longer, died in 1374. William Courtenay, one of Hugh's many younger siblings, was to become bishop of Hereford in 1370, bishop of London in 1375 and archbishop of Canterbury in 1381.

Another nobleman who might have died of plague was Laurence Hastings, earl of Pembroke, who made his will at his Welsh castle of Abergavenny on 24 August 1348 and passed away between 28 and 31 August. Abergavenny lies only a few miles from the Bristol Channel, so it seems possible that one of the many ships sailing into Bristol had carried the infection there. Born in Allesley, Warwickshire in March 1320, Laurence was 28 when he died. He was outlived by his mother Juliana Leyburne, countess of Huntingdon, and his wife Agnes Mortimer, sister of Blanche, Lady Grandison, buried in Much Marcle the year before. Laurence and Agnes's son John Hastings was exactly a year old when he lost his father, and at the age of 11 in 1358 would marry King Edward and Queen Philippa's youngest daughter, 12-year-old Margaret of Windsor.[6] Sir William Hastings, Laurence's illegitimate half-brother and executor, was to die a few months later, and seems likely also to have fallen to the Black Death.

Although the noble, landowning class had more opportunity than others to keep themselves isolated during the pandemic, and thus had more chance to avoid infection, a few high-ranking noble people besides the earl of Pembroke and the earl of Devon's son did die during the plague and perhaps as a result of it. Hugh Despenser, lord of Glamorgan, an important landowner in the south of England and in South Wales – where he owned no fewer than ten castles, including Cardiff and Caerphilly – died on 8 February 1349 at the age of 40. He was a cousin of Edward III, and probably died at one of the many manors he owned in Oxfordshire, Berkshire or Buckinghamshire: the king, then in Kings Langley in Hertfordshire, heard the news of Hugh's death only a day after it happened.[7] If Hugh had died in Wales or in one of his numerous manors in Worcestershire or Gloucestershire, the report of his death would have taken longer to reach Edward. Hugh's tomb and effigy can still be seen in Tewkesbury Abbey in Gloucestershire, lying for eternity next to his wife Elizabeth Montacute (d. 1359), the earl of Salisbury's sister. His effigy shows a clean-shaven, rather handsome man with a short nose and full mouth, wearing a round basinet (helmet) and a tight-fitting leather jupon (a quilted sleeveless jacket) over chainmail and armour. Hugh's cousin Philip Despenser (b. 1313), a landowner in Lincolnshire, followed him to the grave on 22 August 1349, and Philip's mother Margaret Goushill (b. 1294) had died not long before, on *c.* 28 July 1349.[8]

John, Lord Lestrange of Whitchurch in Shropshire died between 13 and 20 July 1349, leaving two sons from his marriage to Ankaret Botiller. The Lestrange brothers were close in age: Fulk, born *c.* 2 February 1331, and John, born *c.* 19 April 1332. Eighteen-year-old Fulk died on 30 August 1349, a few weeks after his father.[9] Alice, Lady Beaumont, titular countess of Buchan and a landowner in Lincolnshire and Leicestershire, died on 9 July 1349.[10] Born in Scotland in the late 1290s, she was the niece and co-heir of John Comyn, earl of Buchan (d. 1308), and in 1310 married the partly French, partly Spanish nobleman Henry Beaumont, who was a great-grandson of the Emperor of Constantinople and moved to England as a child. Alice and Henry's son John Beaumont had been killed jousting in the spring of 1342, and John's widow Eleanor of Lancaster married her second husband the earl of Arundel three years later.

John, Lord Willoughby of Eresby in Lincolnshire died on 13 June 1349. He was 45 when he died, and his son John the younger, born in Spilsby, Lincolnshire on his father's twenty-fifth birthday in early January 1329, lived through the plague. John the son married the earl of Suffolk's daughter

Cecily Ufford and died in March 1372.[11] John and Cecily were the great-great-great-great-great-grandparents of Katherine Willoughby of Eresby (1519–80), who was the daughter of Katherine of Aragon's lady-in-waiting María de Salinas and married Henry VIII's brother-in-law Charles Brandon, duke of Suffolk. And finally, Isabella Verdon, Lady Ferrers of Groby in Leicestershire, was another likely noble victim of the plague, dying on 25 July 1349, aged 32. A great-granddaughter of King Edward I (d. 1307), she was born at Amesbury Priory in Wiltshire on 21 March 1317, eight months after the death of her father Theobald Verdon, and was named after her godmother and great-aunt Queen Isabella, wife of Edward II and mother of Edward III. Her other godmother was Mary, a nun of Amesbury, Edward II's sister. Isabella Verdon and her older half-sisters Joan (b. 1303), Elizabeth (b. *c.* 1306) and Margery (b. 1310) Verdon, came into a sizeable inheritance in the Midlands from their father. At Isabella's manor of Hethe in Oxfordshire, it was said on 27 September 1349 that 'there used to be twenty-seven villeins, but of these, twenty-one are dead and their lands are lying fallow and untilled'.[12]

Chapter 3

The West Country

On 10 October 1348 in Sherborne, Dorset, Thomas Keynes, son and heir of the late John Keynes, proved that he was now 21 years old. He had thus come of age and was old enough to take possession of his father's lands in Somerset, Devon, Hampshire and the Isle of Wight. Thomas was born in his maternal grandfather John Wake's Dorset manor of 'Caundelwake', now called Bishop's Caundle, on 7 July 1327. The 7th of July was the feast of the Translation of St Thomas Becket and was a popular holy day in fourteenth-century England, and Thomas Keynes was presumably named in honour of the saint, the archbishop of Canterbury murdered in his own cathedral in December 1170 (his remains were moved or 'translated' to a newly built shrine on 7 July 1220). A dozen jurors confirmed Thomas's birthdate of 7 July 1327, and gave the reasons why they recalled the date more than twenty years later in October 1348. William Sprot, for example, who was about 60 in 1348, remembered because two days before Thomas Keynes' baptism he had married his wife Joan Hulle in the same church. Three other jurors, who were 55, 60 and 64 years old in 1348, knew the date because they attended the funeral of one William Ivel of Bishop's Caundle on the same day as Thomas's baptism, also in the same church.

Thomas Keynes lost his father at the beginning of 1328 when he was only half a year old, though his maternal grandfather John Wake lived until March 1348, and his mother Isabel Wake was alive during the Black Death and died in 1359. Isabel and her sister Elizabeth Michel, and their 10-year-old nephew John Tyrell, son of their late sister Margery, were co-heirs in 1348 to their father's estates in Dorset and Somerset. A horrifying event of half a century earlier appears in John Wake's inquisition post mortem taken at his manor of Compton Martin in Somerset in March 1348: his mother Alice forfeited the manor in 1299 'by feloniously plotting the death' of Ralph Wake, her husband and John's father. Ralph was poisoned and, according to the inquisition, Alice was punished by being burned alive.[1]

Thomas Keynes survived the first massive pandemic of the Black Death and married a woman called Margery, and their son John Keynes was born in Winkleigh, Devon on 26 November 1352. John had a godmother called Sybil Southcote who was present at his baptism in All Saints' church in the village – the church still stands there today – on the day of his birth, and his nurse was Joan atte Weye. On the day Margery Keynes was purified a few weeks after giving birth to John, her husband Thomas ate breakfast with five residents of Winkleigh, who all recalled the meal more than two decades later. Thomas died at the age of 34 on 29 October 1361, during, and perhaps as a result of, the second pandemic of the plague. His son John Keynes, not yet 9 years old when Thomas died, outlived him by almost six decades and died in January 1420, and Thomas's aunt Elizabeth Michel, one of Isabel Wake's two sisters, was still alive in March 1383.

Thomas Keynes had two cousins via his other maternal aunt, Margery: John Tyrell, born in Rodd, Herefordshire on 3 February 1338, and Hugh Tyrell, born in Broomcroft, Shropshire on 29 November 1341. Mere children during the first pandemic of Black Death, the young Tyrell brothers survived it, though did not live long lives. John Tyrell died in 1360 at the age of only 22, and Hugh died in 1380 also without children from his marriage to Katherine Planke (see Chapter 13 below). The Tyrell brothers lost their father in January 1343 when Hugh, the younger brother, was only 14 months old, and their mother Margery Wake died a year later. Their paternal grandmother Joan Tyrell and maternal grandfather John Wake looked after them, and during their minority Edward III granted custody of the lands of their inheritance to Reynold FitzHerbert of Berkshire, who died on 8 October 1348.

The Wake/Keynes/Tyrell Family of the West Country

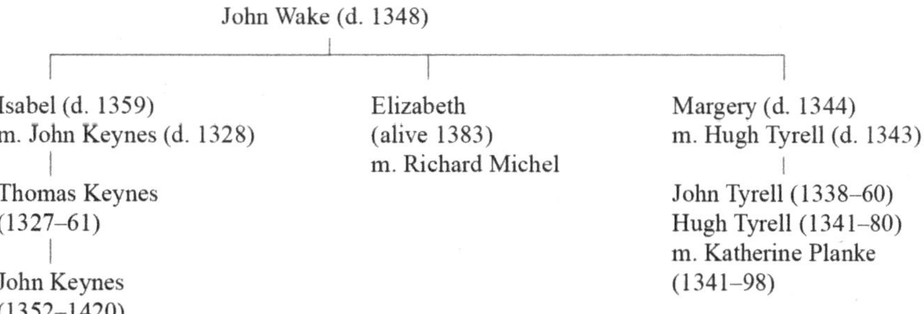

In the summer of 1377, Hugh Tyrell, as constable of Carisbrooke Castle on the Isle of Wight, led a stout defence of the island when it was raided by a force of French soldiers and their allies, the Castilians. He was killed in December 1380 during a military encounter in Brittany.[2]

The fact that Thomas Keynes' proof of age took place on 10 October 1348 in Sherborne, only twenty-five miles from Melcombe, shows that, at least to an extent, life continued as normal several months after the plague's arrival in England. As Benedict Gummer points out, much of Dorset succumbed to the plague that autumn, but, as the county was relatively remote and easy to avoid, the disease progressed only a few hundred metres a day.[3] Twelve men who acted as the jurors, and other officials and administrators, willingly met to confirm the age of a young man who wished to take possession of his inheritance from his late father.

Philip Welleslegh, who held lands in four locations in Somerset including Radstock, and three places in Wiltshire, died on 4 October 1348. Philip's younger daughter Elizabeth Banastre died not long afterwards in her early 20s, leaving a 3-year-old son William; Philip's elder daughter Joan Tudyrleye, about 24 in 1348, survived the plague.[4] The Somerset village of Hinton St George is located thirty miles from Melcombe, fifteen miles from Sherborne and twenty miles from Bishop's Caundle. On 18 October 1348, John Denboud, son of Thomas and Joan Denboud, was born there and baptised by the local parson, Richard atte Hey. Four men of Hinton St George – William Whyte, Thomas Dynham, William Major and Walter Davy – visited Joan Denboud, 'then in childbed', on the day of John's birth. This shows that in fourteenth-century England there was no societal prohibition on unrelated men visiting a woman who had just borne a child while she was still in bed recovering, and also that they had no fear of infecting her with the plague, or perhaps had no concept that such a thing might even be possible. Three other local men went hunting with Thomas Denboud on the day that his son was born and dined with him afterwards in his home, and there is nothing to indicate that anyone in the village feared the plague yet. Thomas Denboud died on 1 January 1362 when his son John was 13, and John's mother Joan was probably already dead then as there is no record of her receiving widow's dower.[5] John Denboud died on 22 October 1390, four days after his forty-second birthday, leaving his widow Margaret and their 18-year-old son John (d. 1429).[6]

Richard Warre, son of John and Joan Warre, had been born in Hinton St George the previous year, on 19 May 1347, and was named after his godfather Richard Blaneford in Hinton church on the day of his birth. Agnes Denboud, grandmother of John Denboud – who would be born in the village just under eighteen months later – was Richard's godmother. Richard lost his father John Warre on 9 May 1349, ten days before his second birthday, at the height of the Black Death, and he himself was still alive in the late 1360s. During Richard's long minority, his family's house, seventy-six acres of land and three acres of meadow were taken care of by locals John and William Beynyn.[7]

Another young person in Somerset who lived through the plague and was a neighbour of the Denboud and Warre families was Joan Chasteleyn. She was born in Dinnington one and a half miles from Hinton St George on 12 March 1348, ten months after Richard Warre and seven months before John Denboud. Joan's father Thomas asked his friend William Welde, then in his mid-20s, if he would act as Joan's godfather. William did not wish to, because he had feelings for Isabel, Thomas's wife and Joan's mother. If he outlived Thomas Chasteleyn, he might wish to marry the widowed Isabel, and becoming her daughter's godfather would create a familial bond between them that would make this impossible. One assumes that William came up with another excuse rather than stating the real reason to Thomas's face. John Vincent, another neighbour who was 18 years old in 1348, did agree to become Joan's godfather. Thomas Chasteleyn had hired Nicholas Cadebury to build a hall in his house in Dinnington and Nicholas showed up for work the day after Joan's birth. In the meantime, Thomas went hunting with his friend John Bruyn, and they 'killed a doe with their bows and arrows'.[8]

Joan Chasteleyn's uncle John Cantelowe owned a house, a garden, a meadow, a mill and seventy-six acres of land in Chilton Cantelo, fifteen miles from Dinnington, and died on 23 March 1349 when his elder daughter Emma, born in Chilton Cantelo on 27 October 1339, was 9 years old. Emma married Walter Park of Upton Scudamore in Wiltshire in or before December 1355, and her younger sister Margaret Cantelowe became a nun at Amesbury Priory in Wiltshire in March 1356. Walter Park died on 4 October 1361, by which time his wife Emma was already dead. The couple were perhaps, as Thomas Keynes perhaps also was, victims of the second pandemic of the plague in 1361. Emma Park née Cantelowe had no children, and her nearest living secular relatives were her cousins Joan Chasteleyn of Dinnington, who was still alive in June 1372 and married to Robert Wyke, and Andrew Homere, who was still alive in 1386.[9]

John Inge of Corston, close to Bath in the north of Somerset, died on 4 February 1349, and his son Andrew died as well sometime before 30 June that year. John's younger son Stephen, said to be 21 months old on 30 June 1349, must also have died not long afterwards.[10] William Tour, born in Broomfield north of Taunton on 29 June 1313, owned a house with twenty acres of land and a meadow close to Broomfield, and lost his father Hugh in May 1321. William was 36 when he died on 28 September 1349, and had a daughter called Alice, who was about 15. Alice married John Roche or Roches on Monday, 8 June 1349, during the Black Death and under 4months before her father died. They had a child before 11 February 1351.[11]

Elizabeth Salmon née Seyncler (or Sinclair), widow of Robert Salmon, died in Chickerell, Dorset on 10 October 1348, the same day that Thomas Keynes proved his age thirty miles away. Chickerell is barely three miles from Melcombe, so Elizabeth might have died of the Black Death. She left a son, John Salmon, who was 5 or 6. Elizabeth was the eldest of four sisters, and her mother Edith Seyncler née Walsh was the youngest of four sisters and had one brother, Nicholas, who was born around 1308. Elizabeth must have been a young mother, as her younger sisters were born in *c.* 1332, 1336 and 1338, and she might not have been much past 20 at the time of her death. Her cousin Simon Brit, son of her mother's sister Maud, was born in Stogumber, Somerset on 18 October 1333, and her cousins Joan and Elizabeth Walsh, daughters of her mother's brother Nicholas, were born in *c.* 1337 and 1338. These two girls would also die during the Black Death (see Chapter 20 below). Elizabeth's son John Salmon was alive in November 1366, and not yet married.[12]

John Aleyn of Purse Caundle, three and a half miles from Bishop's Caundle, died on 4 August 1349, so survived for a year after the plague arrived in Melcombe just twenty-five miles from the cottage where he lived with his wife Isabel and their daughters Eleanor, who was about 6 in 1349, and Joan, who was about 2. Isabel, Eleanor and Joan were all still alive in May 1350.[13] Richard Chambernoun, a child who lived through the plague, was born in or close to Suddon Grange, Somerset and baptised in nearby Wincanton on 29 June 1344. He was named after his great-grandfather and godfather

Richard Lovell of Castle Cary, who was born sometime before June 1276, also survived the horrific first pandemic of the Black Death and did not die until January 1351. Richard Lovell held a celebratory feast several days after his great-grandson's birth at Marsh Court, Wincanton, and evidently was fond of holding feasts to celebrate the births of children: he had done the same thing when William Montacute, future earl of Salisbury, was born in Donyatt in June 1328. His great-grandson and godson Richard Chambernoun was alive in the late 1360s.[14]

In North Cadbury in Somerset, six miles from Wincanton, Isabel Botreaux née Moeles died on either 19 or 20 July 1349, her husband William died on 22 July and her mother-in-law Elizabeth Botreaux died on 20 July. Three members of one family died within two or three days, and Isabel's aunt Margaret Moeles had also died in early March 1349. Isabel and William's son William Botreaux the younger was born in Lanreath, Cornwall on 13 September 1337, and was only 11 years and 10 months old when he suffered the unimaginable trauma of losing both his parents and his grandmother mere days apart. William survived the pestilence and died on 10 August 1391, and his widow Elizabeth Daubeney, rather remarkably, lived until May 1433.[15] Elizabeth was perhaps a good bit younger than her husband, though she was old enough to give birth in *c.* 1367 and must have been past 80 when she died. At the time of her death, she had a grandson who was 43 years old.

In Frome fifteen miles from Wincanton, Andrew Braunche died on 5 April 1349, presumably a victim of the Black Death. Born in Frome on 7 July 1311, son of Nicholas and Robergia, Andrew was 37 when he died, and was a household retainer of Henry of Grosmont, earl of Lancaster, Leicester, Derby and Lincoln. Andrew left a baby son called Thomas Braunche, barely a year old in April 1349.[16] Andrew had married a woman called Joan Kyngeston by October 1335, though his son Thomas was not born until 1348, and perhaps Thomas was the son of Andrew's second wife: there is an undated petition in the National Archives relating to the annulment of Andrew and Joan's marriage.[17] There is no record that Andrew's widow was alive past 1349, and it may be that their son was orphaned at just a year old. Thomas Braunche survived the plague but sadly did not live into adulthood, and died on 20 August 1360, aged 11 or 12. Despite his youth, he was already married to a girl called Mary at the time of his death.

His heir was his much older cousin Stephen Wynslade, born in *c.* 1331, whose mother Eleanor was Andrew Braunche's sister. Eleanor's husband Richard Wynslade died in June 1355, and the couple owned seven houses and over 300 acres of land in and around Frome. In 1355 the houses were said to have been unoccupied and to have fallen into disrepair as a result of the pestilence. Richard Wynslade and Eleanor Braunche's son Stephen died on 18 December 1404, aged about 73.[18]

A Devon woman who survived the plague and lived a very long life was Margaret Hydon, who was born sometime before April 1278 as the only child of Richard Hydon and Isabella Fishacre. Margaret married Joce Dinham in or before 1292, and their first son John Dinham was born in Nutwell, Devon on 14 September 1295; a second son, Oliver, followed before Joce died in March 1301. Margaret married a second husband, Gilbert Knovill, and in 1324 a third, Peter Ovedale, who was many years her junior, born in 1290. Margaret Hydon became a grandmother when her daughter-in-law Margaret, wife of her elder son John Dinham, gave birth to Joan Dinham in late May or early June 1311. John Dinham was only 15 years old when he became a father. The Dinham family were friends with the Braunche family, above: after Andrew Braunche was born in Frome on 7 July 1311, his father Nicholas sent a messenger to young John Dinham, who had recently become a father for the first time. The messenger arrived when John and his wife Margaret were holding a feast to celebrate both her purification after childbirth and the feast of the Translation of St Thomas Becket that day.[19]

The Dinham Family of Devon

Margaret Hydon (before 1278–1357) m. 1) Joce Dinham (*c.* 1273/75–1301)

- John (I) Dinham (1295–1332)
  - Joan (b. 1311)
  - John (II) (1318/19–83)
- Oliver (I) Dinham (*c.* 1297/1300–42)
  - Oliver (II) (1325–51)
    - Oliver (III) (b. 1345, d. before 1357)
    - Margaret (b. 1347) m. William Asthorp
    - Ellen (b. *c.* 1349), nun
    - Isabella (b. *c.* 1350), nun

Margaret Hydon's great-granddaughter Margaret Dinham was born in Hemyock, Devon on 20 July 1347, and her younger sisters Ellen and Isabella Dinham were born during the Black Death in *c.* 1349 and *c.* 1350. Margaret, Ellen and Isabella's older brother Oliver (III) Dinham must have died young, perhaps in the pestilence. Margaret Hydon was still alive to see her great-grandchildren; she outlived her third and much younger husband Peter Ovedale by more than two decades, outlived both her sons, her grandson Oliver (II) Dinham, and great-grandson Oliver (III) Dinham, and lived through the Black Death. She finally died in May 1357.[20]

Joan Lovell, née Ros, died on 13 October 1348 when she must have been in her mid-70s or more; she was old enough to give birth in 1288. Joan outlived her grandson John Lovell (b. 1314) by almost a year, and her granddaughter-in-law, John's widow Isabel, died on 2 July 1349, probably in Sparkford in Somerset, eight miles from Yeovil. Isabel left two young sons, born in 1341 and 1342, who, most confusingly, were both called John. The elder one died unmarried in July 1361, and the younger one lived until 1408 and was the great-great-grandfather of Richard III's friend Francis Lovell, who features in the well-known rhyme 'The cat, the rat, and Lovell our dog/ Rule all England under a hog'. The Lovells' main manor was Titchmarsh in Northamptonshire, a few miles from Kettering, and in February 1351 it was said that 'there were eight bond tenants before the pestilence, of whom four are still alive'.[22]

The Lovell Family of Northamptonshire

John Lovell (I) (d. 1310) m. Joan Ros (d. 1348)
|
John Lovell (II) (1288–1314) m. Maud Burnell (d. 1341)
|
John Lovell (III) (1314–47) m. Isabel Zouche (d. 1349)
|
John Lovell (IV) (1341–61)
John Lovell (V) (1342–1408) m. Maud Holland

Edmund Stonor was born in Ermington, Devon on 28 September 1343, the grandson of John Stonor of Oxfordshire (*c.* 1281–1354), chief justice of the court of common pleas. John the chief justice, his son John the younger and his grandson Edmund all lived through the Black Death, though John Stonor the younger, Edmund's father, died on 31 July 1361 during the second pandemic. Edmund, who died in 1382 in his late 30s, served as sheriff, MP and JP, and was an ancestor of the later Stonor family, who, like the Pastons of Norfolk, are well-known thanks to the large number of letters they wrote that still survive.[23]

The Dorset village of Owermoigne is only eight miles from Melcombe, yet a good few of its residents survived the pandemic of the late 1340s. Henry Moigne was born there on 11 November 1328 and was named after his godfather Henry Sherard, born in *c.* 1290, whose daughter Edith was born in March 1328 and was alive in December 1350, as was her father. William Hamond, Thomas Taillour, Henry Smedmor and John Warmwelle were some of the other village residents alive in 1350. After Henry Moigne lived through the Black Death, he married a woman named Joan Veel and they had a son John, born in Owermoigne on 28 May 1354. They also had younger sons Henry and William and daughters Elizabeth, Agnes and Edith. Joan Veel's mother Katharine Clivedon, Henry Moigne's mother-in-law, married Thomas, Lord Berkeley (d. 1361) of Berkeley Castle in Gloucestershire as her second husband in 1347, and in 1384 founded a school in Gloucestershire that still exists, Katharine Lady Berkeley's School in Wotton-under-Edge. Henry Moigne died on 24 November 1374, aged 46.[24]

On 27 June 1349, William Montacute, earl of Salisbury, proved his age in Somerton, Somerset: he was born in Donyatt, 16 miles from Somerton, on 19 June 1328. His father William Montacute the elder, earl of Salisbury and a great friend of Edward III, was born in Oxfordshire in 1301 and was killed jousting in January 1344, and his mother was Katherine Grandison, who had died two months earlier on 23 April 1349. William's grandmother Elizabeth Montacute née Montfort, who was old enough to bear the eldest of her ten children in the mid or late 1290s, lived through the Black Death and did not die until 1354.[25] In 1349, William was going through an annulment of his marriage to Joan of Kent, a cousin of Edward III, who had committed bigamy and who preferred to be married to her other husband, Sir Thomas Holland. Having lost his father to jousting in early 1344 when he was only 15, and his mother perhaps to the Black Death, William Montacute lived through the horrible experience of killing his only son while they were jousting against each other in 1382. He died shortly before his sixty-ninth birthday in June 1397.

On 2 July 1349, five days after the earl of Salisbury's proof of age, Simon Craucombe died, and his inquisition post mortem was held in Somerton on

20 July. Simon lived in Crowcombe, twelve miles west of Bridgwater, and the Black Death hit the village hard; most of the inhabitants were said to be dead in July 1349. Simon had no children but had a 16-year-old niece called Iseult, daughter of his late younger brother, whose name was also Simon.[26]

Chapter 4

Gloucestershire and Worcestershire

Roger Maltravers, who owned a house and a few acres of pasture and meadow in Little Shurdington between Gloucester and Cheltenham, died on 14 December 1348.[1] This was perhaps a natural death rather than the plague, given Roger's age; his older brother John Maltravers was born in 1266, and Roger's heir was his nephew, John's son John the younger. John Maltravers the son was said to be 60 years old in 1348, which sounds about right; he was old enough to be knighted in 1306 and would have been at least 16 then.[2] The Maltravers men lived long lives: Roger's brother John died in 1341 at the age of 75, and John's son John the younger lived until 1364, when he must also have been about 75.[3] Roger also died at an advanced age, and although many people in the fourteenth century lived longer than their modern descendants often suppose, not many were old enough to have a 60-year-old nephew when they finally passed away. John Maltravers the nephew (*c.* 1288/90–1364) had a son also called John who died on 22 January 1349, leaving three young children from his marriage to a Welsh woman called Gwenllian (invariably spelt 'Wenthliane' or 'Wentliana' in documents written by English people of the era). John and Gwenllian's little son Henry Maltravers, born *c.* 1 January 1348, died before 8 February 1350, though their daughters Joan (b. *c.* 1342) and Eleanor (b. *c.* 1345) Maltravers survived into adulthood. In East Morden not far from Poole in Dorset, part of which was owned by John Maltravers (d. January 1349), it was said on 16 April 1349 that 'all the tenants are dead through the pestilence'.[4]

The plague was in the Gloucestershire village of Dursley, twenty-five miles from Bristol, by early 1349: John Berkeley, lord of Dursley, died not long before 28 January. His widow Hawise outlived him by a few months and died on 24 May.[5] John's inquisition post mortem says that he died on 3 February, but the writ to hold the inquisition was issued on 28 January, so he must have been dead by then. This error is a common feature of 1349 and is an indication of the chaos that reigned that year; English record-keeping in the fourteenth century was usually far more accurate. The village of Dursley is close to the River Severn and about seventeen miles from the modern suspension bridge where the M48 crosses the river. On the other side of the Severn, only a few miles from Dursley as the crow flies but much farther by road in the fourteenth century, stands the village of Awre, and Philip Baderon died there on 13 March 1349. He was born in 1311 or earlier, as he was at least 21 when his father died in 1332, though his brother – or perhaps half-brother – Robert was a good bit younger, born in *c.* 1325. Robert Baderon lived through the pestilence and became a father to Maud in *c.* April 1352 and Joan in *c.* October 1353. He died on 11 October 1361 during the second pandemic.[6]

Nicholas Gamage, who owned a house near Westbury-on-Severn in Gloucestershire, died on either 28 January or 4 February 1349, shortly after John Berkeley of Dursley. He was in his early or mid-40s, and his three daughters, 20-year-old Margery Billing, 16-year-old Joan Arthur and 9-year-old Elizabeth, later called FitzHugh, were all alive in the 1360s.[7] Another Gloucestershire resident was William Lodelawe, which means Ludlow, the town in Shropshire where William or his family must have originally come from. William lived in Chipping Campden and died on 20 May 1349. His son Thomas was not yet 5 years old at the time of William's death, and was alive in 1365.[8] John More of Oldland in Gloucestershire, under 21 years old and still a minor, died on 12 July 1349, though his sister Cecily, born on *c.* 26 December 1334 and 14 at the time, survived and was married by 15 February 1350.[9]

The Wilington Family of Gloucestershire

Ralph Wilington (d. before 1294) m. Juliane

John (d. 1338)
Ralph (d. 1348)
m. Eleanor (d. 1349)

Henry (executed 1322)
Henry (*c.* 1314–49)
John (1340–78) m. Maud
Isabel (*c.* 1370–1424) m. William Beaumont
Ralph (*c.* 1371–82) m. Joan Warre
John (*c.* 1374–96)
Margaret (d. before 1396) m. John Wroth

Eleanor Wilington, widow of Ralph Wilington, a landowner in Gloucestershire, Berkshire, Devon and Cornwall, died on 20 July 1349. Her husband had died fifteen months earlier in April 1348, and Ralph's cousin Henry Wilington (born *c.* 1314) died between 11 and 23 May 1349. Henry's father and Ralph's uncle, Henry Wilington the elder, had been hanged in 1322 in the aftermath of a baronial rebellion against Edward III's father Edward II. Henry the younger's son John Wilington, 9 years old in 1349, was heir to both Henry and Henry's cousin Ralph, and proved his age in 1361: he was born in the Gloucestershire village of Sandhurst, near the River Severn and the city of Gloucester, on 22 February 1340. His father Henry, then about 26, went hunting with his dogs on the day of John's birth, and took a doe. Walter Brounyng, aged 21, resident of Sandhurst, set off to study in Cirencester the day after John Wilington's birth and baptism, and told the abbot of Cirencester the news, while Robert Passemer, 17 in 1340, remembered John's date of birth because a local mill was demolished when the Severn flooded around the same time. John died in his late 30s in August 1378, leaving four children.[10]

The Kerdyf/Wynecote Family of Queenhill, Worcestershire

Paulyn Kerdyf (d. 1291)
|
William Kerdyf (d. 1309) m. Iveta (alive 1314)
|
Paulyn Kerdyf (*c.* 1278/79–1315) m. Eleanor (d. 1349)

William Kerdyf (1299–1331) m. Margaret	Edward Kerdyf (*c.* early 1300s–69)
Joan Kerdyf (1316/17–49) m. 1) John Wynecote (d. 1343) m. 2) John Hampton (d. before March 1349)	Paulyn Kerdyf (*c.* 1349–before 1395)
Margaret Wynecote (*c.* 1338–49) Elizabeth Wynecote (*c.* 1340–49) Eleanor Wynecote (*c.* 1342–49) Another Wynecote daughter (d. 1349) Elizabeth or Margaret Hampton, m. John Baudrip Iveta Hampton, alive 1395, m. Robert Underhill	

In the Malvern hills in Worcestershire, close to where William Langland the poet grew up, is the hamlet of Queenhill, or Quenehull as it was spelt in the fourteenth century. It lies close to the River Severn between Tewkesbury and Upton-upon-Severn, and in the thirteenth and fourteenth centuries belonged to the Kerdyf or Kerdif family, whose name reveals that they originally came from Cardiff. The men of the family alternated the given names William and Paulyn in each generation: Paulyn Kerdyf died in 1291, his son William died in 1309, William's son Paulyn died in 1315 and Paulyn's son William died in 1331.

Paulyn Kerdyf was born in the late 1270s, and was about 30 when his father died in January 1309 and he inherited the manor of Queenhill. Paulyn's mother Iveta, sometimes also spelt Juetta, was still alive in September 1314.[11] He married a woman called Eleanor, and they had a son, William, born on 13 August 1299 when Paulyn was about 20 or 21, followed by a younger son, Edward, born sometime in the early 1300s and perhaps named in honour of King Edward I (d. 1307), Edward III's grandfather. Paulyn died shortly before 10 July 1315, still only in his 30s, when his two sons were teenagers; his widow Eleanor survived him by thirty-four years and died during the Black Death. Although in the fourteenth century men had to wait until they were 21 to come of age, Paulyn's heir William Kerdyf was, unusually, allowed to take possession of Queenhill in April 1316 when he still only 16 years old.[12]

Despite his youth, William was then already married to a woman named Margaret, and their only child, Joan Kerdyf, was born sometime in the last two months of 1316 or the first few weeks of 1317.[13] During Joan's childhood, her father took part in a rebellion against King Edward II and his over-mighty chamberlain and favourite Hugh Despenser the Younger, lord of Glamorgan. The so-called Contrariant rebellion took place in 1321/22 and ended in victory for the king in March 1322; William Kerdyf, having fought on the losing side, was imprisoned. He was still in prison in October 1325 when he was moved from Berkhamsted Castle in Hertfordshire to Pevensey Castle in Sussex, though was released before Christmas that year. William, understandably, supported the revolution against Edward II in 1326/27 that put Edward's 14-year-old son Edward III on the throne, and was restored to his lands by Edward III's mother Queen Isabella, who ruled England during her son's minority.[14] Another dramatic coup took place in October 1330 when Edward III removed his mother from power and began ruling his own kingdom but William Kerdyf did not live long enough to experience much of the young king's governance: he died shortly before 18 March 1331, still only in his early 30s. His wife Margaret outlived him, though for how long is not clear, and she was dead by 1349. Their daughter Joan, aged 14, was given possession of Queenhill in September 1331; in the 1300s girls came of age at 14 if they were married, and Joan was already wed to John Wynecote.[15]

Although she married in her early teens in or before 1331, Joan Wynecote née Kerdyf did not give birth to her first child until *c.* 1338. This was Margaret Wynecote, whom Joan presumably named after her mother, and who was followed by three younger sisters: Elizabeth in *c.* 1340, Eleanor in *c.* 1342 and another little girl whose name and age are unrecorded. Joan was only in her 20s when her husband John Wynecote died not long before 2 April 1343 and left her a widow with four young daughters. The Kerdyf/Wynecote family's overlord at Queenhill was Laurence Hastings, earl of Pembroke (d. late August 1348), and he appointed himself as the four girls' legal guardian, as was customary.[16] At some point, Joan married a second husband, John Hampton, and had two more daughters with him whose names were Iveta and either Elizabeth or Margaret (confusingly, this child bore the same name as one of her older Wynecote half-sisters).

The Black Death was to strike hard at the Kerdyf/Wynecote family of Queenhill. Joan Kerdyf died on Thursday, 12 March 1349 at the age of 32. Her second husband John Hampton was already dead, though the date of his death was not recorded, and he was perhaps also a victim of the plague. In fourteenth-century England, primogeniture – the system of inheritance where the eldest son receives everything – did not apply to female heirs, and Joan's six daughters from her two marriages were entitled to equal parts of her estate. Ten days after Joan's death, Edward III gave custody of the share of her lands that belonged to her eldest daughter, Margaret Wynecote, along with the right to arrange Margaret's marriage at some point, to his servant Thomas Moigne. On 20 April, King Edward claimed that 'some persons have taken away the daughters and heirs' of Joan Kerdyf. In an era when the king owned the marriage rights of underage heirs, for relatives to hide children away to prevent the king from exercising his rights over them was a not uncommon occurrence. In the middle of the greatest pandemic in English history, Edward III, remarkably, sent men to no fewer than eight counties – Worcestershire, Gloucestershire, Oxfordshire, Leicestershire, Warwickshire, Herefordshire, Shropshire and Staffordshire – and instructed them to find the young girls and take them to Gloucester Castle.[17] Three of the Wynecote girls, Margaret, Eleanor and their sister whose name is unknown, died between 12 March and 10 June 1349 and were specifically stated to have 'died in the pestilence'.

Elizabeth, the second eldest Wynecote daughter, outlived her three sisters for a little while but also died on 22 June 1349, or possibly on 1 August. Something of the utter confusion in England in that terrible year of 1349 is apparent first from the wildly varying dates of death frequently assigned to plague victims and second from the inquisitions held to determine the fate of the Kerdyf/Wynecote/Hampton family and who rightfully owned Queenhill after the four Wynecote girls were dead. By English inheritance law of the era, the manor should have been divided between Joan Kerdyf's two young Hampton daughters, who both, unlike their four older half-sisters, survived the Black Death. The heir, however, was first named as Joan Kerdyf's uncle Edward Kerdyf, born in the early 1300s, the younger son of Paulyn (d. 1315) and Eleanor, and brother of William (d. 1331). On another occasion in 1349, the rightful heir was said to be a 60-year-old relative named William Bunynton, who does not otherwise appear on record as a member of the family and was never mentioned again. Edward Kerdyf must have become a father in around 1349: when he died in 1369, probably in his late 60s, he left a 20-year-old son, Paulyn, who died childless sometime before 1395.

To add to the confusion, a woman who died on 10 June 1349 and was named Eleanor was wrongly stated to be the widow of John Hampton, though Hampton certainly married Joan Kerdyf, widow of John Wynecote. As this Eleanor held part of the manor of Queenhill in dower, it seems highly probable that she was in fact Joan Kerdyf's grandmother, the widow of Paulyn Kerdyf (d. 1315) and mother of William (1299–1331) and Edward (d. 1369). Joan Kerdyf's two daughters with John Hampton, either Elizabeth and Iveta or Margaret and Iveta, half-sisters of the four Wynecote girls who died in the Black Death, were later, correctly, named as rightful co-heirs to Queenhill. This younger Elizabeth, or possibly Margaret, eventually had a daughter named Agnes Baudrip and grandsons John and Thomas Basset, while her sister Iveta married Robert Underhill, had no children and was still alive in 1395.[18] These two little girls, who must have been mere toddlers in 1349, were incredibly lucky to survive a terrible disease that took the lives of their mother Joan Kerdyf, possibly their father John Hampton, their four Wynecote half-sisters and their great-grandmother Eleanor Kerdyf within mere months.

Chapter 5

Shropshire and Herefordshire

In the Shropshire village of Alveley between Bridgnorth and Kidderminster, Roger Howell and Thomas Alvedele were both born on 7 July 1348, and Richard Fulybrok, who was 23 years old, married Agnes Fillilode. The following day, another wedding took place in the village when Katherine Solrugge married William Weston. Happily, all these people survived the plague.[1] In the tiny hamlet of More, deep in the Shropshire countryside, John More was born on 8 July 1348, and a few weeks later, on 1 August, 25-year-old William Munede married Agnes Donefow in More. William survived the plague, as did his neighbours Hugh Pursel (born *c.* 1319), Richard Flemmyng (b. *c.* 1315) and Edward Walcote (b. *c.* 1321). William Munede married his second wife Joan Whitton in May 1375, and was still alive in May 1376 in his early 50s.[2] Little John More, born in July 1348 when the Black Death arrived in England, lost both his father William More and his grandfather William More the elder in 1349: William the grandfather died on 10 May and William the father on 22 July. John's mother Elizabeth née Scot survived and was still alive in October 1359.[3] William Pycheford, who owned two houses and land in More, died on 20 July 1349, though his wife Joan and their 6-year-old daughter Alice seem to have survived.[4]

In Much Wenlock, Shropshire on Wednesday, 8 October 1348, two days before Thomas Keynes proved his age 140 miles to the south in Sherborne, twelve jurors met to confirm that John Giffard had also now come of age and was born in the village of Sheinton, three miles from Much Wenlock, on 4 October 1327. His godfathers were Thomas Forcer and John Constantin, who were 44 and 50 respectively when they appeared at the proof of age in the autumn of 1348. Two of the other jurors were Malcolm of Sheinton and David of Drayton, which were both rather unusual given names in fourteenth-century England and were much more common in Scotland.[5] John Giffard's father, also John Giffard, was lord of 'Weston Underegge' in Gloucestershire, later called Weston-sub-Edge, and John inherited a twelfth-century fortified manor-house in the village called Giffard's Manor, which was inhabited until as late as 1800 when it was demolished.[6]

A girl called Alice Rokhull was born on 8 August 1344 in Rockhill, now Rockhill Farm, about four and a half miles east of Ludlow in Shropshire. She was baptised in the nearby village of Greete and named after Alice Parsones, one of her two godmothers. A local couple called William Yonge – who was indeed young at 15 years old – and Joan Stoke married in Greete church on the same day. Alice Rokhull was the daughter of Philip Rokhull, and was the heir of Peter Rokhull, who died on 26 April 1349, and Sibyl Rokhull, who died on 6 July 1349. Peter and Sibyl were either her paternal grandparents or her aunt and uncle. Alice, not yet 5 years old when she lost her relatives in the Black Death, was alive in 1367 and in possession of an acre of land in Rockhill.[7] Another child called Alice from the same area who survived the plague was Alice Carpenter, born in Greete on 10 September 1341 as the youngest daughter of Hugh Carpenter, who died on 18 July 1349. Alice had three older sisters called Margery, Agnes and Isabel, who were all said to be 23 years old in 1358. It is not impossible that they were triplets: in Yorkshire in August 1345, Richard Veile's wife (her name is unrecorded) gave birth to three sons.[8] Margery, Agnes and Isabel Carpenter, alive in 1358, were all dead by late 1365, leaving Alice as Hugh's only living child. One wonders what killed three women who had lived through the plague of 1348/49 that took their father; perhaps they were victims of the second pandemic in the early 1360s.[9]

Joan Stoke, who married William Yonge, had a brother named William Stoke, who died either on 12 or 25 July 1349, six days before or seven days after Hugh Carpenter. The Stoke family owned eighteen acres of land in Greete called *Huntelond*, and it was inherited by William Stoke's son Nicholas. Nicholas was born and baptised in Burford – the village in Shropshire, not the town of the same name in Oxfordshire – on 11 November 1341, two months after Alice Carpenter was born barely two miles away in Greete.[10] Nicholas Stoke's godmother was Margery Boure, whose husband Hugh Boure was one of the coroners of Shropshire and still active in the mid-1370s, when he was said to be 'too sick and aged' to continue working.[11] Hugh must have reached a good age by then, as in 1329 he was old enough to be the godfather of John Halughton, son of Henry and Agnes Halughton. John was born in 'Occleye' or Oakly in Bromfield parish, three miles northwest of Ludlow, on

25 April 1329, and baptised in Bromfield church. John Halughton's mother Agnes, eldest of the four daughters of Philip of Greete, died on 10 August 1349.[12] The Stoke family presumably lived in or close to what is now called Stoke Court, a Grade II* listed building a mile outside Greete, and another resident of Stoke was Simon Cook, who died on 29 September 1349.[13]

The manor of Greete was held by the Cornwall family. Geoffrey Cornwall (d. 1335) was a son of Richard Cornwall (d. 1297), himself an illegitimate son of Richard, earl of Cornwall, the younger brother of King Henry III (r. 1216–72) and uncle of Edward I (r. 1272–1307). Geoffrey married Margaret Mortimer of Richard's Castle on the border of Shropshire and Herefordshire, who was born in 1295 and died in 1345, and their son Richard had a son named Geoffrey after his father. The younger Geoffrey Cornwall was born in Stapleton, Shropshire on 8 September 1335 – the year when his namesake grandfather died – and was baptised in nearby St Andrew's church in Presteigne (which still exists) close to the border of England and Wales. His grandmother Margaret Cornwall née Mortimer sent for the abbot of Wigmore, Richard Turpeton, to act as Geoffrey's godfather. Geoffrey Cornwall survived the Black Death, but his mother Sybil died on 22 May 1349. Geoffrey's first son Brian Cornwall was born on 3 May 1355 in Stokesay Castle near Ludlow, and the long-lived Hugh Boure of Greete took part in Brian's proof of age in Ludlow on 15 May 1376.[14]

Roger Bromleye of Roughton in Shropshire, four miles northeast of Bridgnorth on the way to Wolverhampton, died on 29 September 1349; he left one child, 12-year-old Joan, born around Easter 1337. Roger owned a ruinous house and a small piece of sandy land, said in 1349 to be worth only 2 shillings a year 'because of the pestilence'. Robert Say of Moreton Say near Market Drayton died on 1 August 1349, and his son Robert the younger, born in the village in May 1341, survived. Robert's wife Margaret also survived and married a second husband, Matthew Fouleshurst, before 10 February 1350. Margaret owned an orchard in Moreton Say called *Ympeorchart* or 'sapling orchard'.[15]

Alan Cherleton of Harcourt near Stottesdon in Shropshire died on 1 May 1349, outlived by his father Alan Sr, who died in December 1360, his 9-year-old son John and a younger son, Thomas. Alan Cherleton Jr was 30 years old or under when he died during the pestilence: Nicholas Seymour, the first husband of his mother Ellen Zouche (born *c.* 1288), died in December 1316, and Ellen was married to his father Alan Cherleton the elder by January 1319. Ellen was the daughter and co-heir, with her younger sister Maud, to their father Alan Zouche (1267–1314).[16] Alan Cherleton Jr's first son John Cherleton was born in Prestbury near Cheltenham on 12 March 1340, and was eighteen days younger than John Wilington (see Chapter 4 above), who was born 10 miles away in Sandhurst on 22 February 1340. The same dozen jurors took part in both men's proofs of age on 4 and 18 March 1361, and as is often the case with medieval documents, the jurors' stated ages varied considerably: Hugh Wyneard managed to be 42 years old on 4 March 1361 but 48 just two weeks later, John Theodolf was 57 years old on 4 March but 52 on the 18th, and John Mattesdon was 38 years old on the 4th and 44 on the 18th.

The Zouche/Cherleton Family of Shropshire and Gloucestershire

Alan Zouche (1267–1314)

Ellen (b. *c.* 1288)
m. 2) Alan Cherleton Sr (d. 1360)

Maud (*c.* 1290–1349) m. Robert Holland (d. 1328)

Alan Cherleton Jr (*c.* 1319–49)

John Cherleton (1340–80) m. Joan Langley (1342–68)
Thomas Cherleton (d. 1387)

By March 1359, the month of his nineteenth birthday, John Cherleton was married to Joan Langley, who was then 17 years old. Something soon went wrong between them, however: two years later, John complained that a man named John Trillowe and his associates had abducted his wife from Milcote near Stratford-on-Avon in Warwickshire – Milcote was part of Joan's own inheritance – and had stolen his goods there. By October 1362, Joan Langley was married to John Trillowe instead, and her marriage to John Cherleton must have been annulled. John Cherleton died on Christmas Day 1380, aged 40. His estranged wife had died in October 1368 at the age of 26, and her nearest living relative was a third cousin. According to an inquisition taken decades later in 1409, Joan died pregnant by John Cherleton after they were reconciled. John seems not to have married again, and had no surviving children; his heir was his younger brother Thomas (d. October 1387).[17] John and Thomas Cherleton's great-aunt Maud Holland née Zouche, born in *c.* 1290 and the younger sister of their grandmother Ellen, died on 30 or 31 May 1349, perhaps a victim of the plague, though it is also possible that she died naturally.[18] Maud's son Sir Thomas Holland (born *c.* 1315) married Edward III's cousin Joan of Kent, who in 1349 was in the process of annulling her bigamous other marriage to William Montacute, earl of Salisbury.

Elizabeth Northgrove (or Norgrove), only child of William and Joan Northgrove, came from the Herefordshire village of Tarrington between Hereford and Ledbury. She was born there on 8 September 1345, and was named after her godmother Elizabeth atte Pyrie and probably also in honour of her paternal grandmother, also Elizabeth Northgrove. Her father William, born in *c.* 1318, died in the Black Death shortly before 13 July 1349, when Elizabeth was not yet 4 years old. Her mother Joan not only survived the pandemic but lived for another forty-six years after losing her husband, finally dying in August 1395. Elizabeth also survived the plague, and around 1360 married Robert atte Rydyng, with whom she had children Katherine, Maud and William. She inherited a house in Tarrington with seventy acres of land, and another six acres in *Wynmullehull* (Windmill Hill) in Norgrove, part of the manor of Feckenham in Worcestershire.

The Northgrove Family of Tarrington, Herefordshire

Alvered Northgrove (d. 1302) m. Margery
|
John Northgrove (1297–1320) m. Elizabeth
|
William Northgrove (*c.* 1318–49) m. Joan (d. 1395)
|
Elizabeth Northgrove (1345–78) m. Robert atte Rydyng
|
Katherine (early 1360s–before 1428) m. Richard Beaumont (d. 1428)
Maud (*c.* 1365–1444) m. Richard Avenell
William (*c.* 1367/68–82)

Elizabeth died on 28 November or 1 December 1378, aged 33 and apparently already a widow, though Robert atte Rydyng is oddly obscure, and the date of his death was not recorded. Unusually, Elizabeth always appears on record with her maiden name, not her married name, and as a widow was called simply 'Elizabeth Northgrove' not 'Elizabeth, late the wife of Robert atte Rydyng, daughter and heir of William Northgrove' as would have been customary; in the fourteenth century, women were generally identified by their relationship to their father, husband or brother. Elizabeth's son William was sometimes called by his father's last name, and sometimes by his mother's. He died in 1382, aged 14 or 15, and his older sisters Katherine and Maud outlived him by many years; Maud married Richard Avenell, who came from Much Marcle, eight miles from Tarrington. Elizabeth Northgrove's mother Joan outlived her daughter, her son-in-law Robert atte Rydyng and her grandson William, and Elizabeth's middle child Maud Avenell also lived a long life and died on 29 June 1444, when she must have been close to 80.[19]

Chapter 6

Wiltshire, Berkshire, Oxfordshire

Christina Berenger, who inherited several manors in Hampshire and Wiltshire, died on 12 September 1349. Her age and date of birth are not known, but her brother John – who died in infancy – was born in June 1341, and she was probably within two or three years of his age and was certainly under 14 when she died. Christina was the daughter of John and Emma Berenger, and lost her father in 1343.[1] In 1318, when he was only about 14 years old, John Berenger had raped a young woman named Elizabeth Percy née Hertrigg, who was also 14 or 15, in her father-in-law's home in Great Chalfield, Wiltshire. He was said to have been 'committed to a certain keeper for safe keeping' in July 1319 before he stood trial.[2] Christina's mother Emma married a second husband, Edmund Hakelut (d. 1360), and lived until 1380. Christina Berenger had a half-brother, Leonard Hakelut, who was said to be 11 years old in 1360 and 28 in 1380, so must have been born around the time she died or not long afterwards.[3]

Other Wiltshire victims were the Heyras family from the village of Alderbury, in the south of the county close to Salisbury. Eleanor Heyras died on 28 April 1348 before the Black Death arrived in England. Her 7-year-old son William and her mother Maud almost certainly did die of the plague, however: Maud died on 21 August 1349, and her young grandson just three days later, on 24 August. The heirs to the family's home and five acres of land were Eleanor's sister Joan Harnham and their 13-year-old nephew Robert Pypard, son of their late other sister, Agnes. Robert Pypard was born in Alderbury on 24 April 1336 and named after his godfather Robert Gerard. At his proof of age, four jurors stated that they knew his date of birth because they had been in church hearing Mass during his baptism, and another said that while he was visiting Agnes and her husband John Pypard, their daughter Joan Pypard told him she had a brother just born and baptised.[4]

Just outside Hungerford, close to the border of Berkshire and Wiltshire, Robert Hopegras or Hopgrass owned a house with eighty acres of land, three acres of meadow, seven and a half acres of pasture and thirty-three acres of woodland. The place was later called Hopgrass Farm, and in the twenty-first century is a Grade II listed building just off the A4. Robert and his wife Margery bought the land in 1332.[5] They had a son called Richard, who was about 24 in 1349. Robert Hopegras died on 7 June 1349, and his son Richard died just six days later, on 13 June. Margery is not recorded as receiving her rightful widow's dower, so she was perhaps also a victim of plague, or had died before 1349. William Hopegras, who was Richard's son and Robert and Margery's grandson, and was just 6 years old in 1349, survived the plague.[6] Presumably his mother, whose name is unrecorded, or another relative, survived and took care of him.

William Hopegras spent the rest of his long life in Hopgrass, and was mentioned in the inquisition post mortem of Hugh Stafford, earl of Stafford, in April 1387. On 23 April 1388, when he was about 45, William attended the baptism of one Thomas Lovell in the church of the Holy Cross in Ramsbury, five miles from his house. On his way home afterwards, an unfortunate accident befell William when he fell from his horse in a stony lane and broke his shin. Evidently close to indestructible, William soon recovered and lived to tell this tale at Thomas Lovell's proof of age in October 1409 when he was 66 years old, though he did complain about the pain he had suffered ever since.[7]

In the last decades of the 1300s and well into the 1400s, William Hopegras was active in local government in Wiltshire. In the poll tax records of 1377, there were 75 taxpayers in William's manor, then called Charlton by Hungerford, and the name of one of the tax collectors was recorded as William Hopcroft, perhaps an administrative error for Hop(e)gras(s).[8] William sometimes served as a juror in inquisitions post mortem, and witnessed several grants to Thomas, Lord Berkeley (b. 1353) of Berkeley Castle in Gloucestershire. Lord Berkeley's wife Margaret Lisle (d. 1392) inherited land close to Hopgrass, which Berkeley held until his death in July 1417.[9] William Hopegras was alive in September 1417, when he was named in Lord Berkeley's inquisition post mortem, and dead by June 1423, when his son John Hopegras, who had moved to Dartford in Kent, quitclaimed William's lands in Hopgrass. William's widow Edith was alive in December

1423.[10] A child who survived the first pandemic of the Black Death when he was 6, and all the later fourteenth-century pandemics as well, lived well into his 70s, and might even have reached 80 years old.

William Wantyng was born in Eastbury in Berkshire, between Swindon and Newbury, on Monday, 6 January 1337, and was baptised in the church in Lambourn (then called 'Chepynglambourne' or Chipping Lambourn) two miles away. His parents were John Wantyng and Elizabeth Winterbourne, and he had a sister, Joan, who was probably younger than he. Elizabeth Wantyng née Winterbourne, who came from Wiltshire, died when her son William was 2 years old, and her widower John married a second wife whose name was, like Elizabeth's daughter, Joan. John Wantyng was born in *c.* 1297, and married Elizabeth Winterbourne in or not long after June 1329.[11]

John Wantyng died not long before 13 June 1349, aged about 52.[12] His widow Joan, his 12-year-old son William and his daughter Joan all survived. William Wantyng proved his age in August 1359, but died on 28 October 1361 at the age of 24, possibly a victim of the second pandemic of the plague. He was outlived by his sister Joan, who 'at the time of his death was broken down and of unsound mind on account of a chance illness which attacked her a short time before the death', and their maternal uncle Thomas Winterbourne outlived William too. Another resident of Eastbury was John Grave, who died on 6 February 1349, and an unnamed tenant of John Grave's, who paid 7 shillings a year to live in a cottage in the village owned by John, was said on 27 July that year to be 'dead in the pestilence'.[13]

The village of Broughton Giffard near Melksham had already suffered earlier in 1349 when a flood caused by the endless rain of the last few months submerged eight acres of meadow and, on 30 August 1349, John Arundell was one of the few people still alive in the village after the Black Death. Tidworth is thirty miles from Broughton Giffard and close to the Hampshire border. Sir Henry Husee, who owned part of the manor of Tidworth, died on 21 July 1349, though his wife Katherine survived, and the assignment of dower to her reveals that Tidworth had an east gate and a west gate, two granges, a pigsty called *Hoggehouse*, gardens called *Southgardin*, *Estgardin* (east garden) and *Laurencesgardin*, buildings called *Hyvehous*, *Chafhous* and *Pressourhous*, and a field called *Maydenesdene*. On 26 September 1349, it was said that 'all the tenants are dead' in Tidworth; they included Henry Levechild, John Jaket, Peter atte Nasshe, Walter atte Lidegate, Giles Lylemot, John

Fesaunt, Thomas atte Halle, Henry in the Lane, Simon Norman, William Skynnere, Domenic the smith, the peculiarly and mononymously named 'Cristemasse', i.e., 'Christmas', and women referred to only as 'the widow of the shepherd', 'the widow of Copyn' and 'the widow of Boy'. Tidworth eventually recovered from its terrible losses, and today is best known as a garrison town, with Tidworth Camp, a large Army site, located nearby.[14]

Peter Botiller, lord of Basildon near Reading in Berkshire – not the town in Essex also called Basildon – died on 4 May 1349. At his inquisition post mortem held a month later, it was found that he had once had 100 shillings a year in rent from bondmen and cottars, 'but now all their tenements are in the lord's hands through the death of the tenants during this pestilence and the tenements are worth nothing, for almost all the people are dead this year'.[15] In Stanford in the Vale in Berkshire (now in Oxfordshire), Reynold FitzHerbert, who held the inheritance of the Tyrell brothers John and Hugh during their minority (see Chapter 3), died on 8 October 1348. His toddler daughters, 3-year-old Margaret and 2-year-old Elizabeth, were joint heirs to his house and pasture lands. Reynold was not yet of age in February 1335, therefore, must have been born after February 1314, and was in his early 30s or younger when he died. His older brother Matthew FitzHerbert survived the plague and died childless in December 1356, and Reynold's daughters Margaret and Elizabeth also inherited their uncle's lands in Hampshire, Gloucestershire and Yorkshire.[16]

Thomas Coudray of Lyford and Padworth in Berkshire (Lyford is now in Oxfordshire) died on 16 May 1349, and his widow Joan died on 17 June 1349. One of their tenants, Joan, widow of John atte More, died shortly before 4 June, and another, Thomas Bishop, died on 25 June. Thomas Bishop left daughters Elizabeth, aged 13, and Alice, aged only 2. Thomas and Joan Coudray had a son, Fulk, who was somewhere between his mid-20s and mid-30s in 1349 and was still alive in 1367. According to an inquisition of 20 June 1349, almost all the inhabitants of Padworth were already dead in the pestilence by then.[17] The town did, however, eventually recover, and in the twenty-first century has a population of a little over a thousand.

Sir John Burghersh, owner of the Oxfordshire manor of Ewelme and numerous other estates, died on 29 or 30 June 1349, mere weeks after his wife Maud née Kerdiston died on 20 May. Their heir was their son John Burghersh the younger, who, born in Ewelme on 29 September 1343, was not yet 6 years old when he lost both his parents. On the day of John's birth in 1343, John the father went hunting with a local resident named John Beek, who fell from his horse and broke a leg, and was still lame nearly a quarter of a century later. Seven other residents of Ewelme, all men in their twenties, set off on pilgrimage to Santiago de Compostela together on the day of John's birth. John the son, having survived the Black Death, died in his late forties in September 1391, leaving daughters Margaret, aged about 15, and Maud, aged about 12, from his marriage to Ismania Hanning (d. 1420).[18] Maud Burghersh married the poet Geoffrey Chaucer's son Thomas Chaucer (b. *c.* 1367). It was the Chaucer family's great good fortune that Geoffrey's wife Philippa Roet had a sister, Katherine Swynford, who had a long-term relationship with Edward III's son John of Gaunt, duke of Lancaster, and in 1396 became his third wife. This family connection to one of the most influential men in the country helped to ensure that Geoffrey and Philippa's son Thomas made an excellent marriage to an heiress and became a knight and an important landowner. His and Maud Burghersh's only child and heir Alice Chaucer, born in the early 1400s, became countess of Salisbury by her second marriage and duchess of Suffolk by her third.

Thomas Meaux was born in Bampton, Oxfordshire on 29 January 1349, 'in the first pestilence' as jurors remembered it in 1370. James Moschet died in the town on that day and must have been an infant, as his father John Moschet was only 19; perhaps the little boy was a victim of the plague, though the horrifically high infant mortality rate in the fourteenth century might also be an explanation. Thomas Meaux's godparents were Thomas Boule, vicar of Bampton, Thomas More and Katherine Laundels. He lost his father John when he was young, though his paternal grandfather, Thomas Meaux the elder, lived until 1361.[19]

The hamlet of Tusmore north of Bicester was said in 1357 to be 'void of inhabitants since their death in the pestilence'.[20] In Stanton Harcourt in Oxfordshire, seven of the thirteen villeins on the manor 'died from the pestilence' before 7 November 1349, and in Kidlington in the same county, six of the fourteen bondmen working on the manor were dead by 20 September. Hugh Plecy or Plescy, lord of Kidlington, born in 1319 or 1320, died on 2 September 1349. His heir was his younger brother John, aged about 17, who died at an unrecorded date before he reached 21. Hugh's widow Elizabeth, sister Eleanor, mother Millicent and stepfather Richard Stonlegh survived.[21]

Chapter 7

Surrey, Hampshire, Middlesex

The Grymstede family of Brockenhurst in the New Forest were early victims of the plague: Thomas Grymstede died on 31 January 1349, his brother John on 16 March and their mother Margery on 26 March. The brothers must still have been young: Thomas the older brother was not yet 21 years old in May 1346. Their uncle Peter Grymstede, about 50 years old, lived through the pestilence and was alive in September 1350.[1]

Thomas Horewode of Hampshire died, or perhaps was killed on active service, in Calais on 5 October 1347, shortly after Edward III captured the port. Thomas's parents William and Christiana Horewode survived him but died during the Black Death: William on Monday, 18 May 1349, and Christiana on Saturday, 23 May 1349. William Horewode had been closely associated in the 1320s with Edward II's notorious chamberlain and co-ruler Hugh Despenser the Younger (whose eldest son Hugh, lord of Glamorgan, also died in 1349), though managed to survive Hugh's catastrophic downfall and execution on the orders of Edward II's wife Queen Isabella in 1326.[2] William, Christiana and their son Thomas's heir was Thomas's son William the younger, said to be not quite 7 years old when his grandparents died, and therefore born in *c.* June/July 1342. Thomas's widow Margaret, mother of young William, was granted custody of her son's inheritance on 22 May 1349, the day before her mother-in-law's death, including Polhampton and Stevenbury (part of the village of Preston Candover). Having lost his father and his paternal grandparents before he turned 7, William Horewode finally died on 9 April 1422 at almost 80 years old.[3]

Eleanor Bluet, widow of William Breaunzoun (or Brianzun) and John Bluet, died in Silchester, Hampshire on 28 October 1348. As William, her first husband, had died all the way back in 1310 in his 20s, Eleanor must have been in her 50s or 60s in 1348, and her death was perhaps a natural one, not the plague. She left a daughter, also Eleanor, who was about 30 in 1349 and married to Edmund Baynard, and a grandson named Peter

Cusance, son of her late elder daughter Margaret. Peter Cusance was born in 'the town of St Pancras by London' on 7 February 1329, and proved his age in St Pancras in February 1350, when twelve jurors of the town who had recently lived through the Black Death were summoned to give their reasons for recalling Peter's date of birth. They included Geoffrey Goldbetere, born *c.* 1294, Peter atte Gate, born *c.* 1290, Ellis Bruere, born *c.* 1302 and John Sherewynd, also born *c.* 1302, who remembered the date of 7 February 1329 because he promised to marry Alice Cotesmor on that day.[4]

Joan Wyke of Worplesdon near Guildford in Surrey died on 24 July 1349. Her son Peter Wyke also died in the Black Death, though the date was not recorded; he was alive on 10 March 1349 and dead by 28 March 1350. Peter and his wife Maud had three daughters: Katherine, born in Worplesdon on 20 November 1334 and baptised in Ash, six miles away; Joan, born on *c.* 24 June 1337; and Christine, much younger than her sisters, born on *c.* 12 March 1348. Although the three Wyke girls were alive in March 1350, they then disappear from written record, as does their mother Maud.[5] Richard atte Welle of Compton, three and a half miles from Guildford and seven miles from Worplesdon, died on 26 May 1349 when his son, also Richard, was barely 6 months old. The younger Richard was still alive in 1384.[6]

Sir William Hastings was the half-brother of Laurence Hastings, earl of Pembroke (1320–48), being the illegitimate son of Laurence's father John, Lord Hastings (1286–1325). There is much evidence that William and Laurence were close: Laurence gave William some of his manors in Surrey, Kent, Suffolk, Berkshire, Herefordshire and Wales when he came of age in the early 1340s, they often appear on record as brothers, and William acted as Laurence's executor in the few months between his brother's death and his own. William Hastings passed away sometime between 9 and 23 March 1349, most probably also a victim of the plague. He had no children, and his nephew, Laurence's 18-month-old son John Hastings, was heir to his manors. One of them was Paddington in Surrey – not the area of London with this name – where on 16 April 1349 it was stated that all William's tenants there 'are now dead, except ten'. In William's Berkshire manor of Newbury also on 16 April, an inquest spoke of 'certain free tenants, now dead' who used to pay a total of 40 shillings a year in rent. A tenant of William's in Paddington was Reynold Fulfenne, who had a 3-year-old son named John and died on

22 August 1349, and another was Thomas Sidlesham, who died on 4 May 1349 and had a 2-year-old son also called Thomas.[7]

In Tottenham in Middlesex, Nicholaa Mockyng, daughter of John and Mariote Sterre and widow of the fishmonger John Mockyng, died on 26 September 1348, just under a year after her husband died in early October 1347. Nicholaa and John had three sons and three daughters. Their eldest son John died before his father. Their eldest daughter Felicia outlived her father but died before her mother, and may have been a victim of the plague. Their second son Thomas, about 12 or 14 years old in 1348, outlived his mother by only two weeks and therefore was surely a victim of it, and the same applies to John and Nicholaa's grandson John, son of their late eldest son John, who died between 18 September and 6 October 1348, when he must only have been a small child. Nicholaa's brother Thomas Sterre died in London not long before 26 March 1349, and might also have succumbed to the plague.

John and Nicholaa's youngest son Nicholas, born in the late 1330s, and their daughters Margaret and Idonia, born in the early to mid-1330s, outlived their parents. Nicholas Mockyng was said in an inquisition of the early 1360s to have been 6 years old when his father died in 1347 – though in fact he must have been 8 or 9 – but, despite his youth, he was already married to Margery Malweyn. Nicholas died in October 1360 in his early 20s and, as he had no children, his property passed to his older sisters Margaret and Idonia.[8] Idonia Mockyng, having survived the first pandemic that apparently killed her mother, two of her siblings, her nephew and her uncle, married first John Abyndon and second a draper named Simon Benyngton (d. 1368), who served as one of the two sheriffs of London in the late 1350s. She died in August 1361 in her 20s, and her son John Abyndon the younger died in early 1362; they perhaps both succumbed to the second pandemic of the Black Death. Three shops that Idonia owned in Southwark were said in 1361 to be 'in ruins and without roofs'. Idonia's widower Simon Benyngton married another woman called Idonia as his second wife. In his will of 1368, he asked to be buried alongside Idonia Mockyng in the church of St Laurence in Old Jewry, London, and left money for prayers to be said for Idonia's soul and for those of her first husband John Abyndon and their young son. Margaret Mockyng, the last survivor of her family, married Roger Shipbrok and was alive in May 1372.[9]

John Mockyng the fishmonger (d. 1347) came originally from Somerset and moved to Middlesex, where he and Nicholaa owned 'a third part of a third part' of the manor of Tottenham. They also owned property in London – including a tenement in Pudding Lane, where the Great Fire of London would break out more than three centuries later – and in Great Yarmouth and various locations in Kent. In his will made in September 1347 a month before he died, John divided his property, goods and money among his five living children, including a tavern called *Paulestaverne* (Paul's Tavern) on the west side of Bridge Street in London, which he left to his daughter Margaret. John owned another tavern with an attached shop on the east side of Bridge Street, which passed to his daughter Idonia and was called *Chirchegatetaverne* (Churchgate Tavern) because it was run by William Chirchegate.[10] John had completed his apprenticeship with the master fishmonger Robert Mockyng (d. 1322) in 1311 and, as apprentices sometimes did, took Robert's last name; he was originally called John atte Thorne. The date of his completed apprenticeship suggests he was born *c.* 1290, and was close to 50 when his youngest child Nicholas was born and about 57 when he died in 1347. His father-in-law John Sterre, Nicholaa's father, was also a fishmonger.[11]

Another Middlesex victim was Thomas Duraunt or Durrant (born *c.* 1311) of Enfield, who passed away on 10 May 1349, a few months after Nicholaa Mockyng née Sterre. Curiously, Thomas also had a connection to Somerset, and owned a third part of a manor in the county then called Newton Plecy, later Newton Forester, close to North Petherton just south of Bridgwater. Thomas also owned a 'very well-built' house in Enfield 150 miles east of Bridgwater, which had a garden, two water-mills and a dovecot, and a large amount of land. He had one child, Maud, born in Enfield on 4 March 1338 and 11 years old when she lost her father.

On the morning of his daughter's birth in 1338, Thomas Duraunt met a neighbour, 25-year-old John Tebaud, in church, and invited them to dine with him in his home later that day. Joan Aunsels, one of the women attending Thomas's wife (whose name is not certainly recorded) in labour, 'came running and announced to them the birth of the said Maud'. Another Enfield resident, John Huchon, who was about 45 in 1338 and was still alive in 1353, helped Thomas to catch fish in his fishponds for a feast, to which Thomas invited all his neighbours, to celebrate Maud's birth.

She was named after her godmother Maud atte Merssh ('at the marsh'), and her baptism was conducted by the local vicar, Hervey, who wrote the date and hour in the church psalter. Walter Lorymer of Enfield, born *c.* 1298, stated at Maud's proof of age in 1353 that he 'often heard Thomas, her father, compute the years and days of her age'.[12] On 7 July 1349, Edward III gave custody of Maud's lands, and the right to arrange her marriage, to John Malweyn, whose daughter Margery was already married to John and Nicholaa Mockyng's youngest child Nicholas (who was the same age as Maud Duraunt). By July 1353, aged 15, Maud was married to John Wroth.[13] She had a son named William Wroth, and married a second husband, Baldwin Radyngton or Raddington, who died in 1401. Her son William Wroth died in September 1408, and her grandson, also William Wroth, was born in London on 6 October 1389.[14]

Francis Enefeld, son of John and Margaret Enefeld, was born in Enfield on 25 April 1347, and his godmother was Agnes Duraunt, Maud's mother or grandmother. 'Francis' was a rather unusual name in fourteenth-century England, and was usually spelt 'Frauncеys'. In 1368, some people remembered Francis Enefeld's date of birth because 'the first pestilence happened in those parts in the second year' after he was born. Others remembered it because Edward III's cousin Humphrey de Bohun, earl of Hereford, who was the countess of Devon's brother and was lord of Enfield, 'stayed there at the time of the birth, and on the feast of St. Andrew then next following [30 November 1347] departed therefrom and never returned'. John Enefeld died shortly before 16 November 1349, and his widow Margaret married John Wroth the elder, Maud Duraunt's father-in-law, shortly afterwards on 31 January 1350.[15]

Chapter 8

London (1)

One chronicler says that the plague arrived in London around the feast of All Saints, 1 November 1348, and that, between 2 February and 12 April 1349, over 200 bodies were buried every day in a burial ground next to Smithfield (a number that does not include victims buried in the many dozens of city churchyards).[1] Sir Walter Manny was born around 1310 in Hainault, now a part of Belgium, and was one of the many Hainaulters who settled in England after Edward III married Philippa of Hainault in 1328. Pope Clement VI stated that Walter, 'during the epidemic in England, dedicated a place near London for a cemetery of poor strangers and others, in which sixty thousand bodies are buried'. On another occasion, the pope declared that 'more than sixty thousand bodies of those who died of the epidemic' were buried there. It was known as *Pardonchirchehawe* or 'Pardon Churchyard', which was also the name given to the churchyard of St Paul's on the northwest side of the cathedral. Many dozens of London wills composed during the fourteenth-century plague pandemics requested burial in *Pardonchirchehawe*.[2] The mortality rate among the more prosperous London residents in 1348/49 has been estimated as at least 35% and probably much higher.[3] Of the eight wardens of the guild of cutlers appointed in 1344, all were dead by the end of 1349, and the same applied to all six wardens of the hatters appointed in December 1347.[4] The death rate among the poorer people of London is likely to have been higher still.

Extraordinarily fortunate for English literature, young Geoffrey Chaucer came safely through the plague, as did his parents John Chaucer and Agnes Copton. John was born in London probably in 1312. His father Robert Chaucer came originally from Ipswich and moved to London, where he died in 1315. Robert's wife Mary, John Chaucer's mother and Geoffrey's grandmother, had been married before and had a son, Thomas Heyron, born sometime before January 1305 when Mary was already married to her second husband Robert Chaucer.[5] After she was widowed again in 1315,

Mary married her third husband, Richard Chaucer (who was probably not a relative of her second husband). As a child of about 12 in December 1324, John Chaucer was abducted by his paternal aunt and uncle in Ipswich, who wished to marry him to their daughter, his cousin, to keep property within the family. This soon came to the attention of the authorities.[6] Marrying one's first cousin was all but unknown in fourteenth-century England and, ultimately, John married Agnes Copton instead.

Agnes, Geoffrey Chaucer's mother, was the niece of Hamo Copton, who died in London in the summer of 1331 leaving a son Nicholas, Agnes's cousin. Nicholas Copton appears to have been a victim of the Black Death; he made his will on Saturday, 11 April 1349, during Easter, and died before 27 July. He had a younger half-sister called Mary, daughter of his stepfather Robert Mordon. As Nicholas had no children, and as his half-sister Mary Mordon had no claim to the property of Hamo Copton, who was not her father, Nicholas's cousin Agnes Chaucer née Copton was his heir.[7] Geoffrey's father John Chaucer was heir to his older half-brother Thomas Heyron, who also had no children. Thomas made his will on 7 April 1349, and was already dead when his and John's stepfather Richard Chaucer made his own will just five days later. Richard himself died sometime between 4 May and 20 July 1349.[8] The deaths of Agnes's cousin and John's half-brother during the first pandemic of the Black Death left the Chaucer couple better off than they would otherwise have been. On 13 May 1349, John Chaucer sold his late half-brother Thomas's shop to William Thorney, an alderman of London originally from Lincolnshire, who died before 27 July that year (see Chapter 15).[9]

Sir John Pulteney or Poultney served as mayor of London in 1330/32, 1333/34 and 1336/37, owned a famous mansion in the city called Coldharbour and built Penshurst Place in Kent. On 29 August 1347 in Sutton Valence, Kent, John became the godfather of John Hastings, son and heir of Laurence Hastings and Agnes Mortimer, earl and countess of Pembroke.[10] John Pulteney died on 8 June 1349, though, as he had made his will on 14 November 1348, which in the fourteenth century usually only happened when a person thought s/he might be dying, he might not have been a victim of the Black Death. John was born in or before the mid-1290s, and had moved to London from his native Leicestershire by the mid-1310s.[11] He appointed Laurence Hastings' stepfather William Clinton, earl of Huntingdon (d. 1354), and Ralph Stratford, bishop of London (d. 1354), as supervisors of his will, and gave Stratford 'his finest ring with a great stone called *rubie* of great value and beauty'. Clinton received 'a beautiful ring with two great stones called *diamauntes* [diamonds], two silver flagons enamelled, a cup, together with a certain spoon and saltcellar to match'. John's son William was born sometime between October 1340 and March 1341, survived the plague and died on 20 January 1367, knighted and married but childless.[12] Another former mayor of London was John Hamo or Hamond, a pepperer (spice merchant) who served as mayor from 1343 to 1345. John came originally from Margaretting in Essex, and took his father's given name, Hamo, as his second name. John and his wife Agnes had no children, but he left generous bequests to their nieces and nephews and to Agnes's children and grandchildren from her first marriage to Adam Salisbury (d. 1330). John Hamo died shortly before 2 February 1349.[13]

William Haunsard, who had served alongside John Hamo as sheriff of London in 1333/34 and was a fishmonger by profession, made his will on 6 August 1349 and died before 13 October. His wife Joan of Canterbury also died in October 1349, and their son William Haunsard the younger died before 9 November, two weeks after his mother. The younger William's wife Alice was still alive on 13 October 1349, and he had a sister Margery, then married to Richard Smelt. Margery Smelt née Haunsard was still alive in 1375 and had married a second husband, Richard of Croydon, another fishmonger and perhaps a relative of the fishmongers John (d. 1347) and Hugh (d. 1349) of Croydon. There were two other sisters, Agnes and Isabella Haunsard, who were evidently underage in 1349, as the elder William placed his daughters in the custody of his friend Henry Fanner or Vannere. He also gave Henry and his wife Joan a house in Thames Street.[14]

Thomas Maryns, chamberlain of London – the city's chief financial officer, made his will on 22 April 1349 and died three days later. Thomas qualified as an apothecary after a seven-year apprenticeship in 1310, and as boys usually began their apprenticeship at about 12 or 13, Thomas must have been about 60 years old in 1349. His wife Denise survived him, as did their daughters Margaret and Katherine, the latter a nun at Barking Abbey.[15] Three members of the Shordych family died in quick succession: Robert, warden of the goldsmiths' guild, made his will on 24 March, and was dead by 5 April when his son Edmund made his. Edmund in turn was dead by 17 May when his mother Beatrice, Robert's widow, made her will, and she died before 25 May. Her other sons Simon and Matthew (then spelt Mayhew) were still alive when she made her will. William Shordych, another goldsmith and presumably a relative, as he left a bequest to pay Robert Shordych's debts, made his will on 10 May and died before 20 July.[16]

Isabel Hakeneye grew up near the Tower of London, and cannot have remembered her father, Richard, who died in May 1343 when she was barely a year old. Richard Hakeneye was a *wollemongere*, a seller of wool, one of the two dozen aldermen of London and one of the two city sheriffs in 1321/22. Isabel was raised by her mother, Alice, and her eldest brother Richard the younger; she had another two older brothers, Alan and Neil, and four older sisters, Joan, Lecia, Christine and Pernel. Alice Hakeneye made her will on 15 April 1349, and died before early 1350. Isabel, just 7 years old, had now lost both her parents. Thankfully, her brother Richard survived the pestilence, and was granted official custody of Isabel in February 1350. Isabel married William Olneye (d. 1375), a fishmonger, around 16 August 1362 when she was 20, and they had a son, John Olneye, who died in 1410 while his wife Joan was pregnant.[17]

Old Fish Street (*Eldefisshstrete* in contemporary spelling) was the area of fourteenth-century London where fishmongers practised their trade, and one of them was Roger Bernes. He died in the spring of 1345, leaving a son William, who also worked as a fishmonger and was named after Roger's twin brother, and daughters Joan Braybrok and Roese Bernes. Roger instructed an apprentice named Thomas, who, as apprentices sometimes did, took Roger's last name and was known as Thomas Bernes.[18] By 1349, Roger's son William Bernes was himself instructing an apprentice named William Hedrisham, and had children Benet, Roger, Albreda, Isabel and Juliana.

The Bernes Family of Old Fish Street

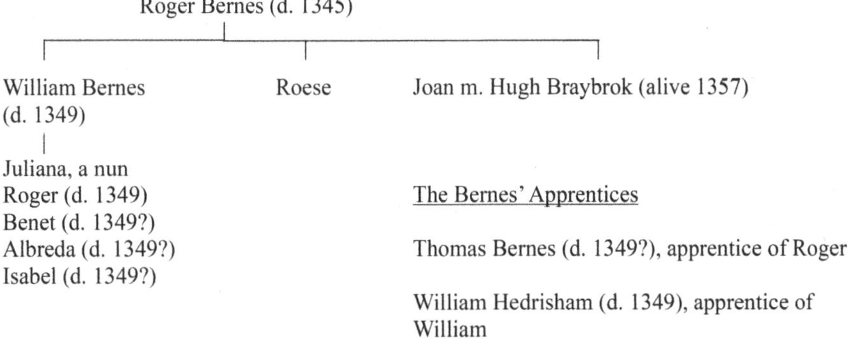

In his will of 8 March 1349, William Bernes appointed his father's former apprentice Thomas Bernes and his own apprentice William Hedrisham as the guardians of four of his children. His other daughter, Juliana, was already a nun, and his wife, whose name is not recorded, was already dead. William Hedrisham made his own will only four days later, and both men died soon afterwards. William Bernes' second son Roger Bernes also died sometime between 8 and 12 March. William Hedrisham, who came from a large family of eight boys and two girls, was still sufficiently *compos mentis* on 12 March to bequeath custody of the surviving Bernes children, Benet, Albreda and Isabel, to John, rector of the church of St Peter Paul's Wharf, where William Bernes and his father Roger Bernes (d. 1345), and probably his son Roger Bernes the younger, were buried.[19] Thomas Bernes, former apprentice of Roger Bernes the elder (d. 1345), almost certainly also died before 12 March 1349, as he does not appear on record again; neither, sadly, do William Bernes' children Benet, Albreda and Isabel, and it seems likely that they died sometime that year while in the rector's custody. William's sisters Joan and Roese were alive when he made his will, and his brother-in-law Hugh Braybrok, Joan's husband, was still alive in May 1357 and living in Enfield in Middlesex. In July 1353, Hugh was one of the jurors who took part in Maud Duraunt's proof of age (see Chapter 7). Hugh was most probably the son of William Braybrok, a fishmonger who was a neighbour of the Bernes family in the late 1310s.[20]

John Palmere came from a family of shipwrights who owned a wharf at Petty Wales near the Tower of London. John was the son of Martin Palmere and the nephew of Alan Palmere, both of whom were master shipwrights, as was John's cousin Philip, Alan's son. John made his will on Wednesday, 7 January 1349, and must have died the same day or early the next day, because, when his wife Amy made her own will on Thursday 8 January, John was already dead. Amy died before 27 July 1349. She and John had a son whom they named Alan after John's uncle, and he was still alive when Amy made her will but might also have died in the pestilence; Amy left money for his care after she died, so he was clearly still a child or an adolescent, but he disappears from record after 1349.[21]

The Palmere Family, Shipwrights of Petty Wales

William Palmere

Alan (d. 1335) — Martin (d. 1344)

Philip (d. 1339) — John (d. 1349) m. Amy (d. 1349)

Alan (d. 1349?)

Adam Aspal worked as a skinner, and in 1344 was appointed as one of the twelve wardens of the guild of skinners. He married Auncilia sometime before October 1339, and they had three children, Juliana, John and Richard. The Aspals paid 60 shillings annually for a house in the parish of St Mary Woolchurch Haw, a church that would be destroyed in the Great Fire centuries later. Sixty shillings was a considerable amount to pay in annual rent in the fourteenth century, even in expensive London, so the Aspals' house would seem to have been a large and well-appointed one. Adam made his will, which mentioned his wife and their three children, on 15 April 1349, and was dead within six days; his sons John and Richard died too in those few days. By the time Auncilia made her own will on 21 April, she had lost her husband and two of her three children, and herself died before 4 May. In her will, Auncilia left money to boys called John and William, sons of the late fishmonger John Neuport, who was perhaps her brother or another relative. The two Neuport boys died in 1349 as well. Juliana Aspal was the only member of the family to survive, and went to live with her 'aunt and next friend' Margaret and Margaret's husband Thomas Thame. This was in accordance with her mother's wishes, and Juliana left the Thame couple 20 shillings in her will.[22] William Cave, one of Adam Aspal's fellow wardens of the skinners' guild, made his will on 7 March 1349 and died before 20 March. In 1341, William had been accused before the Assize of Nuisance of allowing the stone wall of his house near Watling Street to become 'ruinous and on the point of collapse'.[23]

Chapter 9

London (2)

Maud atte Vine of Candlewick Street, who had been taken to the Assize of Nuisance by her next-door neighbour William Peverel on 26 September 1348 after she built an extension on her house that blocked his light (see Introduction above), made her will on 22 April 1349. She died before 4 May. Maud was the widow of John atte Rose, who died before June 1338, and had no children. A well-off, multiple homeowner, Maud left her houses and gardens to her niece Maud Ram, and gave 40 shillings each to her cousins William and Amice Warner. She bequeathed another 40 shillings to the church of Amersham in Berkshire, probably her hometown.[1] Geoffrey Penthog, a *waterlader* or watercarrier, made his will on 30 December 1348, in which he left a garden in East Smithfield to his wife Joan and their son John. By the time Joan Penthog made her own will on 9 January 1349, just eleven days later, her husband and son were already dead, and Joan died before 4 May. She left the garden and the family home to her brother Robert, while the five horses and two carts that Geoffrey had used to transport water around the city were to be 'sold for pious uses' (i.e., the money would be given to charity).[2]

John Neve, a *bureller* (maker of *burel*, a coarse woollen cloth) made his will on 18 December 1348 and died before 1 April 1349; his widow Juliana Neve made her will on 1 April and died before 4 May. She appointed her sister Agnes as her executor. John and Juliana are unlikely to have been a young couple, as in 1326 John was already of an age to be appointed guardian of two orphaned sisters, Margery and Juliana, daughters of the late Elys Chaundeller. Juliana Chaundeller married John and Juliana Neve's son Nicholas Neve, who was a *bureller* like his father, and had a son, William Neve.[3] Roger Syward of Bread Street, also called Roger Peautrer – this meant a person who worked with pewter – was married to Margery, and they had six children born at regular intervals in the 1340s. Margery and all six children were alive in November 1348, but Margery Syward died at an uncertain date in late 1348 or 1349 during the pandemic, and three of her children, John, Constance, and Joan, died before 19 August 1349. Her widower Roger died before 20 July 1349, leaving his and Margery's 6-year-old son William, 5-year-old daughter Marion and 1-year-old son Thomas. Six-year-old William Syward also died not long afterwards, and Marion and her little brother Thomas were given into the custody of their uncle John Syward (d. 1375). Another of the late Roger's brothers, William Syward (d. 1368), also appears to have looked after his orphaned niece and nephew. Marion was alive in 1358 and Thomas was alive in 1367, the only survivors of what had been, until the end of 1348, a family of eight. Constance and Joan were younger than their sister Marion so cannot have been much more than toddlers when they died in the Black Death, and John, eldest of the six Syward children, was well under 10 years old in 1349.[4]

The Syward Family of Bread Street

Roger Syward aka Roger Peautrer (d. 1349) m. Margery (d. late 1348 or 1349)
|
John (*c.* 1341/42–49)
William (*c.* 1343–49)
Marion (b. *c.* 1344, alive 1358)
Constance (*c.* 1345/46–49)
Joan (*c.* 1346/47–49)
Thomas (b. *c.* 1348, alive 1367)

Roger Carpenter, son of Thomas (d. 1336) and Alice Carpenter, worked as a pepperer, and married a woman with the unusual name of Mazera. They had children, Alice, Thomas, Isabella and Agnes; Alice, the eldest, was in her teens and already married by 1349. Roger made his will on 24 March 1349 and died the same day. His stepmother Maud, his wife and his four children were all then alive, but Mazera and their daughters Isabella and Agnes died before Christmas 1349, as, almost certainly, did Maud. Roger and Mazera's eldest child Alice and her husband George Cosyn survived and were both still alive in May 1351. In December 1349, young Thomas Carpenter, the only son, was placed in the custody of a mercer named Thomas Brandone. By then, the boy's only living relatives other than his older sister Alice were his aunt Agnes Chalk and her husband William. He was still alive in 1362.[5]

In his will of 30 January 1349, Stephen Waltham, a girdler (maker of girdles), appointed his wife Margery as one of his executors and left her their house in the parish of St Laurence, but when Stephen died just days later, on or before 2 February, Margery was already dead.[6] The potter John Romeneye made his will on 23 April and died before 4 May, and his widow Agnes, daughter of Alan of Suffolk (d. 1337), made her will on 9 June and died before 7 December.[7] Richard Stokwell of Red Cross Street (then called 'Redecrouchestrete') made his will on 4 April and was already dead when his son Hugh made his on 8 April. Hugh Stokwell died before 4 May, and left his property to his stepmother Alice, Richard's widow, in accordance with his father's wishes. Richard Stokwell worked as a painter, as did Walter Stokwell, who died in 1349 along with almost all his family, and they were probably relatives.[8]

Maud Weston died not long before 6 December 1349. From her first marriage to Robert Raughton, a maker of metal pots, Maud had children Alice, William and Thomas Raughton, and by January 1329 she had married her second husband Peter Weston, also a maker of metal pots, who died in 1347. Maud had another son called Henry, probably Peter's son, and her eldest son William Raughton was, like his father and stepfather, a potter. Maud was outlived by her mother-in-law Katherine, Peter's mother and apparently by all her four children, the Black Death taking a much less heavy toll on the Raughton/Weston family than on many other London families.[9] In 1349, Stephen atte Holte, a timber-monger in Birchin Lane, was a widower with two daughters, Agnes and Maud, and was instructing an apprentice called Richard atte Grove. Stephen died not long before 26 March 1349, and in his will appointed his associate Simon Caproun or Caperon as his daughters' guardian. Agnes, the elder daughter, was just 5 years old in 1349, and her little sister Maud must also have died shortly after their father made his will. Simon Caproun apparently was another victim of the plague, as the London authorities placed Agnes atte Holte in the custody of a carpenter named John Bergholte, not in Simon's. By the end of 1357, although Agnes was still only 13, her guardian had, rather creepily, married her. In 1354, Agnes had been abducted from their home by Richard and Alice Stanford in what was surely an attempt to gain control of the money and goods she inherited from her father Stephen, by marrying her to their son.[10] The marriage was perhaps intended to prevent such an occurrence happening again.

Agnes Fraunceys and her husband Thomas, a wax-chandler (maker of wax candles), who lived in Candlewick Street, died mere days apart in March 1349, though their daughter Marion appears to have survived. Her mother left her a green coverlet embroidered with roses and lilies, silver spoons and 'a robe of gold work'. Ralph and Margaret Merk were another London couple who both died in 1349. Ralph, a fishmonger, had a son called Roger from a previous marriage.[11] John Youn came from a family of fishmongers and was perhaps a nephew or a younger son of Robert Youn, a London fishmonger who died in 1321. John made a will on 11 April 1349, the Saturday between Good Friday and Easter Sunday. He left bequests to his wife Joan, their daughter Joan, who was a nun of Rusper Priory in Sussex, their other daughter Margery, Margery's husband Richard Youn – who took his wife's name – and Margery and Richard's son John. By the time Joan Youn the mother made her will a month later, on 11 May, she had lost her husband, their daughter Margery, their son-in-law Richard and their young grandson John, and Joan herself died before 9 June. The fate of her other daughter Joan the younger, a nun, is uncertain.[12]

The Youn Family of London

John Youn (d. 1349) m. Joan (d. 1349)
|
Joan, a nun, fate unknown
Margery Youn (d. 1349) m. Richard (d. 1349)
|
John Youn (d. 1349)

The Mymmes family lived on the road in central London called Poultry, and consisted of parents John and Maud and their daughters Alice and Isabel. Both John and Maud worked as *ymaginours*, image-makers. Maud described her profession as 'the making of pictures' and instructed an apprentice called Thomas. Evidently an energetic woman of many talents, she also ran her own brewery. John Mymmes made his will on 19 March 1349, and died before 10 April, when Maud made her own will. She died before 25 May. Maud bequeathed 'the third best part of copies and instruments pertaining to the making of pictures, and one of her best chests for keeping them in' to her apprentice Thomas – the two best parts were for her daughters – and arranged for Thomas to continue his training with Friar Thomas Alsham at Bermondsey Priory after her death.

Alice, the elder Mymmes daughter, died sometime after Maud made her will, though Alice's sister, 8-year-old Isabel, survived. John Mymmes had specified in his will that his friend Roger Osekyn, a pepperer, should have custody of his and Maud's daughters if Maud died before they came of age, but Roger died as well in early May 1349. Isabel Mymmes was instead placed in the custody of a man named Thomas Staundone, presumably a relative of her mother Maud, and was alive in 1362 and dead by 1378.[13] Roger Osekyn was himself the second of four sons of Robert Osekyn, a carpenter who died in 1311, and Joan Callere, who died in 1317, and he was still underage in 1319. He was outlived by his brothers John and Simon, and his daughter Joan Osekyn also survived the plague and died in 1392. Although she had married Walter Etecrone, a pepperer like her father, she always used her father's last name.[14]

William Newenham died in London not long before 20 July 1349. He left four children, of whom only one, a son also named William, was legitimate. From a relationship with Agnes Dolfyn, William had an illegitimate daughter called Agnes and, from a relationship with Maud Blaket of Rickmansworth, he had illegitimate children called John and Joan. Agnes must have been older than her three half-siblings, as, in his will, William Newenham appointed her as his other children's official guardian, and she was also William's executor and ultimately his sole heir after her half-siblings died. She married John Bryd, a draper of London, who in 1364 had to seek sanctuary in the church of St Martin le Grand after committing a felony of some kind. His apprentice John Robyn of Hertford asked the London authorities to release him from his apprenticeship, as his master was 'a fugitive' in the church, 'from whence he dare not stir, and accordingly was unable to instruct him in his trade'.[15]

Another resident of London with illegitimate children was John Gildesburgh, a fishmonger, and John and his brother Richard were also of illegitimate birth themselves. John made his will on 17 July 1349 and died on or around 18 October that year. He had three illegitimate daughters with Isabel Moleseye, called Margaret, Isabel and Juliana, who survived the plague and were all still alive in 1361. Thomas Burton, a mercer, died not long before 8 June 1349, and his brother-in-law Walter Costantyn died before 20 July. Walter Costantyn left money to his wife Alice so that she would assist their niece Amice Burton, Thomas's daughter, 'towards her marriage or some trade befitting her position'. Thomas's own very brief will does not mention Amice; he left a house and shops in the unfortunately named Gropecuntelane in London to his associate John Howle or Holegh, a wealthy hosier of illegitimate birth who lived through the pandemic and died in February 1352. John Howle was a member of the family; his second wife Isabel was Thomas Burton's niece and Amice's cousin.[16]

One of the sheriffs of London in 1345/46 was Edmund Hemenhale, a mercer by profession. He made his will on 26 December 1348 and died before 12 October 1349. Edmund's son Thomas was 4 and his daughter Margaret just 1 year old when he died, and they were still alive in the 1360s. Edmund also had a son John, who was mentioned in his will but does not appear on record after 1349, so perhaps also died in the Black Death.[17] John Wynchelseye, a baker, made his will on 24 March 1349 and died before 20 July. His (unnamed) wife was already dead, and he appointed her brother Richard Walssh and Richard's wife Margery as guardians of their daughters Alice and Margaret. The girls also inherited their father's goods, including a silk girdle, a gold bracelet and silver cups and spoons.[18] John Dallyng, a mercer, was one of four brothers and four sisters. He made his will on 6 April 1349, leaving his tenement in Bassishaw ward to his son John the younger. He died before 20 May, when 'the tenement in which my father died' is mentioned in John the younger's will. John Dallyng the son died before 23 November 1349.[19]

A hospital was founded in London in July 1330, and was officially called the 'Hospital of St Mary within Cripplegate'. Its founder was a wealthy mercer called William Elsing or Elsyng, and many Londoners called the place *Elsyngspital* or *Elsinggespitele*, i.e., Elsing Spital. In his will of 24 March 1349, William Elsing specified that the hospital was for the 'poor, blind and indigent of both sexes, under the direction of a prior and convent'. William died in or before early May 1349, and his son Robert, also a mercer, died between June and October 1350. Robert Elsing was married to Alianore, who died before him, and their son Thomas was born in or not long before February 1347. Thomas made his will in March 1430 and died in November 1431, having outlived his parents by more than eighty years. Until he came of age in early 1368, his guardian was his father's cousin, Jordan Elsing.[20] Elsing Spital was closed by Henry VIII, but some remains of it still exist in the twenty-first century on the road called London Wall, near the Barbican Centre and Liverpool Street railway station.

Another London mercer, Roger Pycot, died sometime in 1349 when his sons Thomas, born in March 1346, and Simon, born in May 1347, were toddlers. The boys' mother was already dead and, at the start of 1350, guardians were found for them: Thomas was given into the custody of William Todenham and Simon into the custody of Nicholas Ploket, both of whom also worked as mercers. The Pycot brothers lived into adulthood, and both claimed their inheritance from their father when they came of age at 21 in 1367 and 1368 respectively.[21] John and Alice Northall were the guardians of their grandson John Bonaventure, son of their late daughter Wymarca and her late husband Bonaventure Bonentente of Florence (there was a sizeable Italian population in fourteenth-century London). John Northall made his will on 5 May 1349 and died before 25 May, though his widow Alice lived until 1361, and their partly English, partly Italian grandson was alive in 1367. Wymarca and Bonaventure were married by early 1336, and John was said to be 8 years old when Wymarca died in August 1345.[22]

John Coterel, a mercer of London, had three children from his first marriage to a woman whose name is unknown, and married second a woman called Alice. In 1349, his son Thomas was 2 years old and his other son John was 3, and his daughter Joan was older than her brothers. John Coterel made his will on 3 April 1349 and died before 23 July that year. His two little sons died shortly afterwards as well. His widow and executor Alice survived and was still alive forty years later in the late 1380s and, after her husband's death, continued instructing his apprentice and relative Geoffrey Colewelle. Alice's stepdaughter Joan was also still alive in the late 1380s and married to John Body. In his will of April 1349, Joan's father John Coterel left £40 to his son Thomas, £20 to his son John and £40 to Joan and, as the sole survivor, all of it passed to Joan.[23]

Chapter 10

The Isle of Wight and Sussex

The Black Death reached the Isle of Wight by the spring of 1349, the waters of the Solent proving no barrier to the infection. A sad story of a child from the island who survived the first pandemic of the Black Death in 1348/49, but died in a later one, is that of John Lisle, here called John Lisle III to distinguish him from his father and grandfather of the same name. He was born in his maternal grandfather John de Bohun's manor of Cowdray near Midhurst in Sussex on 6 November 1342, and grew up in his father's manor of Gatcombe on the Isle of Wight with his sister Elizabeth, who was two or three years younger. John and Elizabeth's father, John Lisle II, was born on 13 June 1324. He married Joan de Bohun of Sussex in the late 1330s or early 1340s and was 18 when their son was born in November 1342; Joan was about the same age.

The Lisle Family of Gatcombe, Isle of Wight

Geoffrey Lisle (d. 1293) m. Iseult Albemarle
|
Baldwin Lisle (1270–1307)
|
John Lisle I (1303–37) m. Joan (d. 1349) who m. 2) Henry Romeyn (d. 1349)
| |
| Edmund Romeyn (d. 1349?)
John Lisle II (1324–49)
m. Joan de Bohun (d. after July 1360, daughter of John de Bohun (1301–67))
|
John Lisle III (1342–69) m. Alice (d. 1369)
Elizabeth Lisle (*c.* 1345–after 1402) m. John Bramshott

John Lisle III was not yet 6 years old when the plague arrived in England in the summer of 1348, and he lost his father on 31 March 1349. John Lisle II was still only 24 years old when he died. John III's paternal grandmother, confusingly also called Joan, followed her son to the grave either on 26 July or 27 August 1349. She was the widow of John Lisle I (d. 1337) and was in her early or mid-40s when she died. Joan had married a second husband,

Henry Romeyn, who owned lands and houses in Hampshire and Sussex and died on *c.* 12 May 1349, a few weeks after his stepson John Lisle II. Henry had a son Edmund, who was either 6 or 8 years old in 1349 and might have been Joan's son (and thus the much younger half-brother of John Lisle II), though he might have been born to Henry's previous wife. The date of Edmund Romeyn's death is not recorded, but he did not live into adulthood.

John Lisle III's mother, Joan Lisle née de Bohun, and his maternal grandfather, John de Bohun, survived the plague of 1349, as did his younger sister Elizabeth. As a widow, Joan was entitled to hold a third part of her late husband's lands for the rest of her life, and her third of the manor of Gatcombe was minutely detailed in October 1349. It included 'a low chamber at the west head of the hall', a small building with a wash house and larder, a kitchen and attached dairy, a small chamber at the east end of the hall with another chamber above it and a chimney, a garden called *Uppegardyn*, a small vegetable plot, access to the well, meadows called *Longemede* and *Whitemede*, a wood called *Westwode*, and the rents and services of seven bonded tenants, two women and five men. The list of their names usefully reveals who had survived the Black Death: Isabel atte Shute, Margery Gippes, John Hurlebat, Philip Snotedon, Geoffrey Portesy, Robert Girpe and Thomas Short. It is notable that every one of them was unmarried, suggesting that, at least in some cases, they had had spouses who died of the plague. Another tenant of the Lisle family in Gatcombe was Richard atte Halle, who died on 4 April 1349 four days after his landlord John Lisle II, leaving a 2-year-old son, Robert, who was still alive in 1384. Two other men from Gatcombe who died in the plague were John Hachard and Walter Bretecombe, and John Hachard was a shepherd who lived next to a piece of arable land called *Fisacres*. Some of the people in Cowdray in Sussex, John Lisle III's birthplace in 1342, who survived the first pandemic and were alive in the 1360s were Agnes Stainer and her father Nicholas, John Elkham, John Brokere, Henry Exton, Robert Fauconer and Robert atte Rode.[1]

Joan Lisle née de Bohun's father John de Bohun of Sussex was born in November 1301, and her mother was called Isabel Tregoz. Her brother Edward de Bohun, their father's heir for many years, was his nephew John Lisle III's godfather, and survived the plague of 1348/49, but died in 1361 in their father's lifetime. John de Bohun died in December 1367 at the age of 66, and his daughter Joan Lisle was still alive in July 1360.[2] Her son John Lisle III of Gatcombe died on 3 September 1369, not yet 27 years old, having outlived his maternal grandfather by less than two years. John's wife Alice died the day before he did.[3] It therefore seems highly likely that the young couple were victims of the third outbreak of the Black Death, which struck England that year. As John and Alice had no children, John's heir was his 24-year-old sister Elizabeth, who was married to John Bramshott of Hampshire. Elizabeth had a son, William Bramshott, and among her descendants were the Dudley family, prominent in Tudor times. Robert Dudley, earl of Leicester (1532–88), courtier and favourite of Queen Elizabeth I, was her great-great-great-great-grandson. Elizabeth Bramshott née Lisle was still alive in November 1402.[4]

Another example of a child surviving the first pandemic but dying as an adult in a later one may be found in the Noion family of East Anglia. John Noion died on 2 July 1349 and his wife Beatrice on 12 July, leaving their son John, who was about 4 or 6 years old. John survived the plague in 1349 but died on 14 August 1361, perhaps in the second pandemic, aged about 16 or 18.[5] And another child on the Isle of Wight who did succumb to the plague in 1349 was Margaret Doget, daughter of the late Geoffrey Doget (d. 28 January 1345). She died in Bouldnor near Yarmouth on the island on 7 April 1349, a week after John Lisle II died ten miles away. Margaret, said to be 2 years old at her father's inquisition post mortem in May 1345, was still only 6 when she died. Her heir was her cousin Alice Doget, born *c.* 1336/37, daughter of Geoffrey's brother Walter, and the inheritance comprised a house with forty acres of arable land and nine acres of pasture. In 1353, this land was described as 'late in the hands of tenants', strongly implying that the tenants were all dead in the Black Death.[6]

Eight miles from the Lisle family's home in Gatcombe lies the village of Shalfleet. Its parson during the plague, appointed in April 1348, was John Seys, described as the 'illegitimate son of a married man'.[7] Richard Compton was born in Merston Pagham on the Isle of Wight on 1 February 1346 and was baptised in the church of Arreton, ten miles from Shalfleet, on the day of his birth; his godfathers were Richard Freland, parson of the church of Kingston on the island, and Reynold Hayward. Richard's father and grandfather were both called John Compton. One of them died shortly before 12 March 1349 and the other shortly before 3 November that year, and Margery Compton, Richard's grandmother, also died on 15 April 1349.

Richard, just 3 years old, lost his father and grandparents in the space of a few months. His mother, as there is no record of her alive after 1349, perhaps also succumbed. Her identity is uncertain, though John Compton the grandfather complained in October 1337 that three named men and unnamed others 'took away John his eldest son … [and] married him against his will'.[8]

John Compton the grandfather was born in *c.* June 1298, and was 48 when his grandson Richard was born and 51 when he died.[9] His son John the younger, Richard's father, was probably in his early teens or thereabouts when he was abducted and forcibly married in 1337. In 1346, the year of his grandson's birth, John the elder was arrested and imprisoned in London on a charge of wounding a man in the left hand so that he died, presumably of gangrene or blood poisoning. Edward III, however, declared that John had been 'indicted by malicious procuration'. Four years earlier in 1342, with a large gang of associates, John the elder broke into a house in Merston Pagham, where they stole goods and money and assaulted the servants.[10] His grandson Richard Compton survived the pandemic and was still alive in late 1367 shortly after he came of age, though subsequently vanishes from the record.[11] And two other victims of the plague on the Isle of Wight were Reynold Ogelondre or Oglander of Nunwell, who died on 14 May 1349, and John Heyns of Stenbury, three miles from Ventnor, who died on 4 June 1349. Reynold's son Robert, presumably named in honour of his grandfathers Robert Ogelondre and Robert Urry, was just a month old when Reynold died, and he and his mother, Reynold's widow Roberta, were alive in November 1349.[12]

John Evenyng or Avenyng of Eastbourne in Sussex died on 2 October 1349, and his daughter Isabel, married to Geoffrey Sonnynglegh, died sixteen days later, leaving her baby son John Sonnynglegh, born at Christmas 1348. John Evenyng was said to be about 30 when his father Simon died in 1328, so was in his early 50s when he died. His son-in-law Geoffrey was still alive in the late 1370s, married to a second wife called Joan.[13] William Bonett or Bovett of Wappingthorn in Sussex died sometime before 18 March 1349, his daughter-in-law Margaret died on 24 September 1349 and William's elder son Neel or Nigel, Margaret's husband, was alive on 18 March but died before Margaret. Born on *c.* 19 January 1329, Neel was 20 when he died, and his mother Joan née Combes, who died before the plague arrived in England, was born in about 1309. William and Joan Bonett's younger son William,

Neel's brother, born in March 1336, was still alive in 1358. On 24 March 1350, five freemen and one bondman were alive in Wappingthorn and paid a total annual rent of 12s 6½d; 'other tenants, who brought the rent up to 60s formerly, [are] dead and their holdings stand empty'.[14]

Walter Crulle of Slaugham in Sussex died on 9 April 1349, though his stepson Thomas Thorndenne, then about 37 years old, was still alive in the early 1370s. Walter's neighbour Adam atte Nasshe died two days after he did, and a nobleman, Thomas, later Lord Poynings, was born in Slaugham on 19 April.[15] In his early 20s, Thomas became the third of the five husbands of Blanche Mowbray, daughter of Lord Mowbray. Blanche was a few years older than Thomas, and lived until 1409; Thomas himself died childless in 1375. John Bulsham of Bilsham in Sussex, in the parish of Yapton close to Bognor, died on 1 July 1349. On 21 November that year, 'the tenants [of Bilsham] are all dead ... and no one will rent their tenements or have anything to do with them'.[16] This is perhaps evidence of a kind of superstitious dread, an unwillingness to live in or even to enter a house where people had died of plague.

Chapter 11

Nottinghamshire and Northamptonshire

On 11 August 1348 in Nottingham, Laurence Pavely proved, as Thomas Keynes did two months later in Dorset, that he was now 21 years old and had come of age. He was born in Bingham nine miles east of Nottingham on 25 July 1327, eighteen days after Thomas Keynes was born 200 miles away in Bishop's Caundle. Laurence was now entitled to hold the lands in Nottinghamshire and Northamptonshire formerly owned by his father Robert, who had died in November 1346.

A panel of a dozen male jurors confirmed Laurence's date of birth and gave the reasons why they remembered when he was born. The unfortunate William Gunter, aged about 50 in 1348, recalled the date clearly because his kitchen burned down four days after Laurence was born, Ralph Asshefordby knew it because his brother William got married five days later and John Poigne, aged about 60 in 1348, remembered because his cousin Thomas Bingham was caught in bed with Laurence's nurse a few weeks after the boy's birth.[1] Laurence's grandfather, also called Laurence Pavely, was born in August 1258 as the elder of twin boys. As the elder twin, Laurence inherited the entire Pavely family estate while the younger, Philip, received nothing.[2] Laurence Pavely the younger, born in July 1327, was the eldest of four brothers, and he and his next two brothers died during the Black Death and almost certainly from it (see pages 72–73 below).

In the village of Wiverton in Nottinghamshire, William Cotegrave died on 19 June 1349. He had no children, and his brother Robert was already dead, though Robert left children Margery, Henry, Alice and Cecily Cotegrave, born between the early 1330s and the early 1340s. Henry Cotegrave died in 1354 and his three sisters outlived him.[3] Also in Wiverton, John Knyght died sometime in the early summer of 1349, and another victim in the village was Elizabeth Garthorp, who died on 29 or 30 June 1349.[4] She was only 14 when she passed away, and was outlived by her paternal grandmother Joan, widow of Hugh Garthorp, who died in September 1318 when Elizabeth's father William was about 3 years old.[5] Hugh Garthorp had a sister whose name was also Joan, Elizabeth's great-aunt, who married Joce Spalding of Lincolnshire. The Spaldings moved to London, where they owned a house near St Paul's Wharf and lived next door to Rose Hert, a widow who annoyed them by keeping her pigsty too close to their common wall and causing it to collapse. On the other side, Joce and Joan's neighbour was Hamo Chigwell, a fishmonger who served as mayor of London no fewer than eight times between the late 1310s and late 1320s.[6] Joce Spalding killed a draper named Thomas Kyrkeby in April 1325 after the two men quarrelled in the London church of All Hallows on the Cellar. Thomas chased Joce out of the church, punched him in the face and drew his knife on him. Joce drew his own *anelaz* (dagger) to defend himself, and in the ensuing struggle stabbed Thomas in the chest and killed him. Joce was incarcerated in Newgate prison but not executed, and eight months later Edward II pardoned him on the grounds that he acted in self-defence. He was still alive in January 1338.[7]

The Garthorp Family of Nottinghamshire

Hugh Garthorp (d. 1318)   Joan Garthorp m. Joce Spalding (alive 1338)
m. Joan (alive 1349), who m. 2) Gerard Seckyndon
|
Denise (alive 1349)
Emma (alive 1349)
William (1315–37) m. Maud (d. after 1338)
|
Elizabeth Garthorp (1334/35–49)
Emma Garthorp (1336–*c.* 1340)

In 1319, six years before killing Thomas Kyrkeby, Joce petitioned Edward II for custody of his and his wife Joan's nephew, Hugh and Joan Garthorp's son William, and for the custody of Hugh's house and seventy-seven acres of land in Nottinghamshire. Edward granted the petition and told the Spaldings to maintain William in food, clothing and necessaries, but although Joce and Joan had also asked to be granted William's marriage rights, in July 1321 Edward II sold them instead to Robert Melton of Leicestershire. William's mother, Hugh Garthorp's widow Joan, married her second husband Gerard Seckyndon or Sekynton of Warwickshire before July 1321. Joce Spalding, for some reason, became convinced that his brother-in-law Hugh Garthorp had never been legally married to Joan, now married to Gerard, but failed to convince the authorities of this.[8]

Sometime before 1334, William Garthorp married a girl or young woman called Maud, most probably a relative of Robert Melton, who had bought the rights to his marriage in 1321. Their first daughter, Elizabeth, was born in late 1334 or early 1335 when William was almost 20, and their second, Emma, in late 1336. William was still only 22 when he died shortly before 10 June 1337; Elizabeth was 2 and a half years old when she lost her father and Emma was 7 months. William's widow Maud was still alive in April 1338 but then disappears from the record, and her infant daughter Emma died before July 1340, when Edward III gave Elizabeth Garthorp's marriage rights to Richard Ty, parson of Multon, and did not mention Emma.[9] Elizabeth lost her parents and her sister when she was only a young child, though her paternal grandmother Joan, widow of Hugh Garthorp and Gerard Seckyndon, was still alive.

Fourteen-year-old Elizabeth Garthorp made a will on 29 June 1349, in which she mentioned property in London that she had presumably inherited from her great-aunt and great-uncle, Joan and Joce Spalding. She died either that same day or the day after. She had, of course, no children, and her heirs were her father William's sisters Denise and Emma Garthorp, daughters of Hugh and Joan, who were both said to be over 30 in 1349 and were not yet married.[10]

In Carlton-in-Lindrick north of Worksop, William Fourneux died on 21 August 1349, and his sister Joan FitzHenry died on 15 September. Joan's 10-year-old son Henry FitzHenry, and her and William's nephew Thomas Latimer, son of their late sister Sybil, survived.[11] Laurence Pavely, who was born in Bingham near Nottingham in July 1327 and proved his age in August 1348, died unmarried on 7 June 1349, a few weeks before he would have turned 22. Almost certainly, Laurence died in Paulerspury near Towcester in Northamptonshire, as he was buried in the church of St James the Great in the village. On 28 June 1349, jurors at Laurence's inquisition post mortem found that the Pavely family's manor of Paulerspury, then called 'Westpirie', had until recently been worth over £23 a year in rents from 'free tenants, bondmen and cottars, but they are all dead, except a few'.[12] Laurence's heir was his 20-year-old brother Roger Pavely, but Roger also died sometime between 15 and 28 June 1349, and it seems highly likely that both young men were victims of the plague. Another brother, William, still alive when their father Robert died in November 1346, was by now also dead, and therefore

Laurence's heir was the fourth Pavely brother, John, who was not quite 16 years old. John Pavely was born in Little Houghton near Northampton on 2 July 1333 and, not long after he was born, 'there was a great fire at Little Houghton, and the whole town was almost burnt, and the said John, lying in a cradle, was carried into a field for fear of the fire'. John was confirmed by the bishop of Lincoln, Henry Burghersh (d. 1340), who had come to the village to reconsecrate the church, which had been badly damaged by the fire, and stayed in the home of John's father Robert Pavely. Robert was attending the county court in Northampton Castle when he heard the news that his fourth son had been born, and immediately afterwards travelled to Scotland to join Edward III's army: the king defeated a Scottish force at the battle of Halidon Hill ('Halydonhull' as it appears in John Pavely's proof of age in 1354) on 19 July 1333.[13]

In Great Houghton, a mile from Little Houghton, Brian Saffrey, who owned a house there, died on 21 June 1349.[14] His daughter Alice was 5 years old and outlived her father by only a year: she died on 19 June 1350. Her aunt and uncle, Brian's sister Joan and brother Thomas, survived the plague. Brian Saffrey was born on *c.* 7 July 1314 so was not quite 35 when he died, Thomas was born in *c.* 1316 and Joan in *c.* 1320, and their father William (d. 1325) came originally from Pampisford in Cambridgeshire. Their mother was called Margery Stane and came from Silton in Dorset, though she inherited some land in Great Houghton from her mother Christine Daubeney.[15]

One village in Northamptonshire that disappeared as a result of the pandemic of 1349 was Hale, which lay a few miles south of Apethorpe and west of Peterborough. In 1356, an inquisition stated that 'no one dwells nor has dwelt in Hale since the pestilence', and it is now considered a lost medieval settlement. In Castle Ashby, eight miles east of Northampton, then called 'Assheby David', only six of the twenty-four bondmen of the village were still alive on 26 June 1349.[16]

William Carvaill, who owned a house, sixty acres of arable land and twelve of meadow next to the River Nene in Earls Barton in Northamptonshire – the village where Thomas Swetcok drowned in a pond in 1348 – died on 24 June 1349, three days after Brian Saffrey died seven miles away in Great Houghton. William had three sons, Thomas, John and Robert, who were all alive in 1342 but died before their father, perhaps in the pestilence.

William's youngest and only surviving child was Maud, born in Earls Barton on 27 October 1343. Maud's mother Isabel also died in or before 1349, and she was given in ward to her father's brothers John and Thomas. Before October 1362, Maud Carvaill married Robert Haldenby.[17] In Desborough, fifteen miles from Earls Barton, two cousins born on the same day were growing up during the pestilence. Emma Burdoun and William Geffrey were both born on 22 October 1335 and were baptised on that day in the same church, with the same holy water, two hours apart. Emma's father was Stephen, who died before 20 May 1350, and her mother was Sarra.[18]

Hugh Lutryngton of Hackleton in Northamptonshire, not far from the Buckinghamshire border, died on 2 July 1349, and his wife Joan and their son Richard also died shortly before Hugh did, though the dates of their deaths are not recorded. Richard must have been a young child, as his sister Katherine, who survived the plague but lost her entire family – her paternal uncle, another Richard – also died, was only 4 years old in 1349. She was still alive in February 1360, and had recently turned 15 years old.[19]

Peter Prilly or Purley of Little Oakley, Northamptonshire was probably born in 1318, son of Hugh and Margery Prilly, and grandson of Peter Prilly the elder and Alice Kirkby. Peter the grandfather and his son Hugh died a day apart in November 1322, when young Peter was 4 years old. Young Peter's mother Margery outlived her husband Hugh by many years; she was still alive in November 1344, and was probably the 'Margaret Prilly' who died shortly before 10 November 1349.[20] Sometime in the first half of the 1340s, Peter married Lucy, third and youngest daughter of Guy Mancestre (*c.* 1291–1365) of Mancetter in Warwickshire, and their sons Hugh and William were born just thirteen months apart on *c.* 1 August 1345 and *c.* 8 September 1346. Guy Mancestre was one of the jurors who took part in the proof of age of Laurence Hastings, earl of Pembroke, when Laurence proved in 1341 that he was now 21. Laurence was born in Allesley fifteen miles from Guy's home in Mancetter, and Laurence's mother Juliana sent a messenger to Guy to inform him of her son's birth. Guy had the date inscribed in his psalter.[21]

Peter Prilly died on 28 June 1349, aged 30 or 31. There is no record of his wife Lucy Mancestre receiving her dower, so either she was another victim of the plague, or she had died sometime between September 1346, when her second son was born, and June 1349. As noted above, Peter's mother

Margery or Margaret may also have died in the late autumn of 1349. Peter and Lucy's elder son Hugh died around the time of his twelfth birthday in August 1357, and their younger son William died in May 1393, leaving a teenage son named Peter, who had descendants. The Osevill family of Leicestershire were relatives of the Prilly family: Alice Kirkby, paternal grandmother of Peter Prilly who died in 1349, had a younger sister named Margery, who married Walter Osevill. Margery and Walter's son Hugh Osevill died on *c.* 12 March 1349, perhaps a victim of the plague like his cousin Hugh Prilly's son Peter. As Hugh Osevill's son John Osevill and John's son William Osevill died before him, his heir was his granddaughter, John's daughter Cecily.[22]

The Kirkby, Prilly and Osevill Families of Northamptonshire and Leicestershire

Alice Kirkby m. Peter Prilly (d. 1322)	Margery Kirkby m. William Osevill
Hugh Prilly (d. 1322) m. Margery (d. 1349)	Hugh Osevill (d. 1349)
Peter (1318–49) m. Lucy Mancestre	John (d. 1349 or before)
Hugh (1345–57) William (1346–93)	William (d. 1349 or before) Cecily

Chapter 12

Buckinghamshire, Bedfordshire, Hertfordshire

The wedding of Alice Lenard and William Cok in Chalfont St Giles, Buckinghamshire on 5 September 1348 perhaps indicates that news of the plague had not yet reached their village, 130 miles northeast of Melcombe in Dorset. In the same village on the same day, a boy named Philip Vache was born and baptised, and King Edward and Queen Philippa's eldest daughter Isabella of Woodstock travelled there to act as his godmother. Alice Aleyn was hired as the infant's wetnurse, two women named Alice Cud and Agnes Schulle carried him to the church for his baptism, and Alice's father Thomas Cud was buried in the churchyard also on 5 September: with a wedding, a funeral and a baptism all taking place on the same day, it was a typically busy day for the local parish church. Henry Lenard, whose daughter Alice had just married William Cok, invited little Philip Vache's family into his house after the baptism and 'made him [Philip] warm' – another indication that, at the end of the dismal summer of 1348, it was still so unseasonably chilly and wet that fires had to be lit. Having lived through the greatest pandemic in history in his earliest years, Philip made his will on 25 April 1407 and died before 10 October that year, aged 59.[1]

Another resident of Chalfont St Giles was John Wolverton, who was born around 1295/1300 and died on 13 July 1349. His youngest child was Ralph, just 2 years old in 1349, and he had six daughters as well from two marriages: Joan, Sarah, Cecily, Constance, Margery and Elizabeth, all of whom were much older than their little brother. Joan, the eldest Wolverton daughter, outlived her father by just five days and died on 18 July 1349, and left a son called John Wake who was about 13 years old, eleven years older than Joan's half-brother Ralph Wolverton.[2]

Sir Philip Aylesbury, lord of Newport Pagnell in Buckinghamshire, twelve miles from the Pavely family's manor of Paulerspury in Northamptonshire, and a former sheriff of Bedfordshire and Buckinghamshire, died on 14 July 1349. Philip was also lord of Milton Keynes (Middelton Kaynes, Mideltonekaynes or Mitilton Caynes, as it was spelt at the time), which, despite its image as a town created in the second half of the twentieth century, did already exist as a village in the fourteenth. Philip owned Milton Keynes by right of his late wife Margaret, daughter and heir of Robert Keynes, and they owned a house there with eighty acres of arable land and four acres of meadow. Their house stood near the churchyard and had a room called *knightis chaumbre* or 'knights' chamber' with two adjoining rooms, a dairy (*deyhous*) with a bakehouse next to it, two ponds, two dovecots, a *schephous* (sheep-house) outside the gates, a wood and a water-mill called *Foxesmilne*. Another resident of the village of Milton Keynes in 1349 was Henry Ward, who on 29 March that year was given a house in nearby Broughton by William Withtheberd or 'with the beard'. William was alive on 7 November 1349, though it is not clear if Henry Ward survived the plague.[3]

As Margaret Keynes and her son Thomas Aylesbury were already dead in 1349, the village of Milton Keynes and the rest of Margaret and her husband Philip's lands were inherited by their grandson, Thomas's son John Aylesbury. When Philip died in July 1349, John was 15, having been born in Weldon, Northamptonshire on 6 May 1334. The village of Weldon belonged to John's maternal grandfather Ralph Basset (1300–41), who was also one of John's two godfathers, the other being Warin Latimer. A grandfather at only 33 or 34 years old, Ralph Basset was evidently a man of quick and violent temper: he punched one of his servants, Richard Reve, on the neck when Richard innocently asked him during John Aylesbury's baptism why the infant was not named after one of his godfathers. Rather more happily, Henry Burghersh, bishop of Lincoln, came to Weldon to confirm John Aylesbury, as he had done for John Pavely ten months earlier and twenty-five miles away, and Ralph Basset held jousts at his manor of Weldon a few weeks later to celebrate the purification of his daughter Joan, John's mother. Until he came of age in 1355, John Aylesbury was placed in the official custody of William Clinton, earl of Huntingdon, stepfather of Laurence Hastings, earl of Pembroke. John survived all the pandemics of the Black Death and served, as his grandfather also had, as sheriff of Bedfordshire and Buckinghamshire. In the 1380s and 1390s, he and his cousin John Knyvet spent many years pursuing a claim to be the rightful heirs of another cousin, Ralph Basset the younger, who was murdered in 1385. The two men affected to believe that Ralph's son and heir Richard was in fact the illegitimate son of a man named Tybot Lowekin. John Aylesbury died on 7 December 1409 at the age of 75.[4]

John Aylesbury's godfather Warin Latimer of Braybrooke in Northamptonshire died either on 13 August or 8 September 1349, 'at the end of the pestilence', according to an inquisition held a few years later. Born around 1304, Warin was in his mid-40s when he died and left his widow Katherine (d. August 1361), their daughter Elizabeth and their sons John, Warin, Thomas and Edward Latimer. John Latimer the eldest son was born in *c.* February 1335, and the middle two sons Warin and Thomas were twins, with Warin the elder, born in Braybrooke on 14 September 1341. The family's name often appears as Latimer Bochard or Bouchard, presumably to differentiate them from other families with the common name of Latimer.[5] All five Latimer children, who probably grew up in Braybrooke Castle, a fortified and moated manor-house in Northamptonshire, survived the plague. John the eldest brother died in France 'three months after the taking of King John of France', a reference to the capture of John II of France by Edward III's eldest son the prince of Wales at the battle of Poitiers in September 1356. Thomas Latimer, who held the family's estates after his older brother John and his older twin Warin died, was a Lollard, a follower of John Wycliffe. He died on his sixtieth birthday, 14 September 1401, the day after making a will that began 'I Thomas Latymere of Braybrok a fals knyt [false knight] to God…'. Thomas left no children, and his heir was Edward Latimer (Bochard), youngest of the four brothers, who survived the plague in early childhood and lived until 1411.[6]

Reynold Meleward or Mulward of Sutton a few miles east of Bedford died sometime in 1349, though the precise date was not recorded. He was born shortly before 10 October 1321, so was 27 or 28 when he died, and his son William was 3 years old in 1349.[7] John Exmue of Wymington in Bedfordshire died on 21 June 1349 at the beginning of his 30s. His wife, name unknown, appears to have been already dead, and he left one child, Clemence or Clemency, who was born on the feast of St Clement (23 November) in 1347. John owned a house and dovecot with almost 250 acres of land, which would eventually have passed to his infant daughter when she came of age, but Clemence died on 16 July 1361 at just 13, perhaps in the second pandemic of the plague.[8] John Hervy of Riseley, ten miles north of Bedford, died on 29 June 1349, leaving a house and 300 acres of land, said in July 1351 to be 'unoccupied and uncultivated' after the Black Death, to his 3-year-old granddaughter Athelina Hervy.[9] And Thomas Potyn, a wine merchant, made his will in Little Hadham near Bishop's Stortford on 22 July 1349, and died before 19 October.[10]

Another Brian Saffrey, who must have been a cousin of the Brian Saffrey in Great Houghton, Northamptonshire mentioned in Chapter 11 above and who owned a smallholding and a few acres of 'poor and sandy arable land' in Cainhoe and Clophill in Bedfordshire, died on 28 July 1349. Although he left a 2-year-old daughter called Joan, she must have died young, as Thomas Saffrey, brother of the Brian Saffrey in Great Houghton, was this Brian's ultimate heir as well.[11] Peter Seint Croys or Saint Cross, another landowner in Cainhoe, Clophill and Ampthill, died on 8 April 1349. In Ampthill on 15 May 1349, an inquisition found that 'all the bondmen and cottars are dead through the pestilence', and Peter's son Robert also died on 24 May 1349. Robert Seint Croys was supposedly 24 when he died in May 1349, though on other occasions was specifically said to have died a minor, i.e., under 21 years old. Then again, Robert's son Thomas Seint Croys was said to be 21 years old in July 1362, i.e., he was born in 1341, and it is hard to see how Robert could have been under 21 in 1349 and yet have had a son then 8 years old, and a document from December 1327 that refers to Peter, his wife Margery and their son Robert reveals that Robert had been born by then. Assuming that he was indeed 24 in 1349, he must have become a father at about 16.[12]

In the Hertfordshire village of Sacombe near Stevenage, it was said in October 1352 that 'the tenants are dead, and many lands lie untilled'.[13] In Standon five miles from Sacombe, Thomas FitzEustace died on 3 August 1349. In May 1342 he was 13 years old, so must have been 20 when he died, and had a brother John, who was born in Shenley, Buckinghamshire on *c.* 24 June 1338 and named after his godfather John atte Welle. John FitzEustace died in 1369, during the third pandemic, a few weeks after his son Philip was born.[14] Sixteen miles from Sacombe is the village of Ashwell, and in St Mary's church a famous inscription was carved in 1349: 'Wretched, terrible, destructive; only remnants of the people remain.'[15]

A few miles south of Ashwell and nine miles from Sacombe, the village of Hunsdon was the birthplace of Amyel Honesdon, who worked as a chandler (candle-maker). Amyel died sometime before January 1341, when his wife

Maud née Manhale made a will calling herself his widow and mentioning their daughters Joan, Christine and Margaret. Margaret, the youngest daughter, died sometime between 1341 and 1349, and her sisters Joan and Christine appear to have been victims of the Black Death: Joan died not long before 9 February and Christine not long before 16 February 1349. The wills of the two sisters, who were not married, reveal the fluidity of last names in the fourteenth century: Joan called herself Joan Amyel, their father's given name, and Christine's surname was Chaundeller, their father's profession. They were still underage when their mother made her will in early 1341, so were only in their late teens or early 20s when they died days apart in February 1349.[16]

Alexander and Agnes Mareschal of Luton both died in 1349, Alexander before 23 March and Agnes before 20 July. They had a daughter, Joan, who married Thomas Cotynham and had a daughter whom she named Agnes after her mother. One of the Mareschal couple must have been related to, or had some other kind of close association with, Amyel Honesdon or his wife Maud Manhale, as Amyel and Maud's daughters Joan and Christine both left them property, and Christine Chaundeller asked Alexander to pay her debts and funeral expenses. In his will, Alexander, who was a blacksmith, gave the tools of his trade to his former apprentices Walter and John Halpeny and his current apprentice John Poulsherst, except for his three best anvils and a thousand horseshoes, which went to his wife Agnes. She outlived him by mere months, however.[17]

Another Hertfordshire victim was Amice Polayn of Ayot St Peter (called 'Aiete Mofichet' in her inquisition post mortem) who died on 24 March 1349.[18] People who lived through the plague in the village of Benington, ten miles from Ayot St Peter, and were still alive in 1353 included John Chiltren, born *c.* 1309, his wife Alice and their son Richard, born in 1332; Adam Heron, born *c.* 1305; Henry Melksshop, born *c.* 1299; William Gobyoun, born *c.* 1305; Thomas Chapman, born *c.* 1309; and Walter Revel, born *c.* 1300.[19]

Chapter 13

Leicestershire, Warwickshire, Staffordshire

William Planke, a landowner in Leicestershire, Northamptonshire, Wiltshire and Buckinghamshire, was born in Curry Mallet, Somerset on 2 October 1325, the son and heir of William Planke the elder (early 1300s–35).[1] In or not long after 1336, William married Elizabeth Hillary, daughter of Sir Roger Hillary, chief justice of the courts of King's Bench and Common Pleas. William was about 11 at the time, and Elizabeth was probably a little older. He was a very young father: Katherine Planke, the eldest of his and Elizabeth's three daughters, was born in Bescot, Staffordshire on 6 January 1341 when William was 15 years and 3 months old, and must therefore have been conceived when he was only 14. Katherine was baptised in nearby Walsall on the day of her birth, and her godfather was Thomas, abbot of Hailes Abbey in Gloucestershire. Two of the men present in the church during her baptism recalled a few years later how they saw her carried back home amid 'singing and a great concourse of people praising God for her birth'. Fourteenth-century England was a place where people sang and danced with joy when children, including female children, were born, and after the baptism of John Amory in Frolesworth, Leicestershire in November 1331, he was carried to his parents' home from church 'with the joy of the neighbourhood'.[2] It was also the custom for new parents to provide a meal for their friends and neighbours to celebrate the mother's purification thirty to forty days after giving birth.

Katherine Planke was presumably named in honour of her maternal grandmother Katherine Hillary, and the manor of Bescot, her birthplace, belonged to her Hillary grandparents. Her father William died on 5 September 1347, eleven months after he came of age at 21, possibly as a result of military action during Edward III's wars in France. He died exactly a month before Thomas Horewode of Hampshire (see Chapter 7). William Planke and Elizabeth Hillary had two other daughters after Katherine in 1341: Joan, born in *c.* 1344, and Elizabeth, who was posthumous, born in

Walsall probably on 1 January 1348, and therefore still a baby when the Black Death arrived in England later that year. Joan Planke, the middle daughter, died in Bescot on 1 July 1349 eighteen months after the birth of her little sister, aged about 5, perhaps a victim of the plague.[3]

It is not clear when Elizabeth Hillary, the Planke sisters' mother, died, but the two surviving girls were in the care of their maternal grandparents Sir Roger and Katherine Hillary until Roger died on 1 June 1356 and his widow just nineteen days later. In his will, Roger requested burial in the church of All Saints in Walsall, where his granddaughter Elizabeth Planke was baptised at the beginning of 1348.[4] Roger and Katherine's son and heir Roger Hillary the younger, born *c.* February 1331, then took over custody of his nieces. Soon afterwards on 3 July 1356, Katherine Planke proved that she was now 15 years old and was entitled to claim her half of her late father William's inheritance, with her younger sister Elizabeth due the other half when she came of age. Their middle sister, Joan, would also have been entitled to an equal share of the inheritance had she survived the Black Death. Although Elizabeth Planke was only 8 years old in 1356, she and her older sister were already married to brothers: William and John, sons of Sir Fulk Bermyngham of Warwickshire.

The Hillary/Planke family did not fare as badly in the Black Death as numerous other families did, with Joan Planke and perhaps her mother Elizabeth Hillary the only casualties. Roger Hillary the younger, uncle of the Planke sisters and in his late teens during the pandemic, lived until June 1400 and was buried in the same church as his father in Walsall; his badly damaged effigy, lying on his side, can still be seen there. Katherine the elder surviving Planke daughter married again twice after her first husband William Bermyngham died. Her second husband was Hugh Tyrell, born in Shropshire in November 1341 and a cousin of Thomas Keynes (see Chapter 3 above), and after Hugh was killed in the duchy of Brittany in 1380, Katherine married Bernard Brocas (*c.* 1330–95). She died in October 1398.[5] Her sister Elizabeth, who was born three months after their father died and lived through the first massive pandemic of the Black Death as a baby, had a long and eventful life. She died in September 1423 at the age of 75, having married another three husbands after John Bermingham: Lord Grey of Rotherfield, Lord Russell and the earl of Huntingdon's nephew Lord Clinton. Despite their adventurous marital history, marrying seven husbands between them, neither Katherine nor Elizabeth had any surviving children. Elizabeth's nearest blood relative when she finally died was the great-great-grandson of their father's aunt.[6]

In Leicester, Henry Belgrave was alive on 25 March 1349, and was well enough then to seal a document granting a small plot of land to four associates in exchange for an annual rent of two shillings in cash plus two hens and a cock. He died a few days later, on or before 31 March, when his wife Agnes was described as his widow. Richard Swepston, who lived just outside the North Gate of Leicester, was alive on 29 December 1348 and dead by 25 March 1349. His wife Alice and their son Hugh outlived him, and Hugh was still alive in the late 1360s, as was Richard's brother William Swepston.[7] John Bentley of Bentley near Walsall died on 26 April 1349. Born on *c.* 29 September 1329, John was only 19 years old when he died, and left a 5-month-old son, William, born in Little Saredon near Wolverhampton on 21 November 1348. John's wife Maud appears to have died too, though his sister Ellen survived, and her son William Leche was alive decades later in London. John and Maud's son William Bentley married a woman called Eleanor, and died childless on 6 September 1387.[8]

Between Wolverhampton and Stoke-on-Trent is the village of Eccleshall, and Alice Bromley was born there on 31 October 1347 as the only child of John and Hillaria. John Bromley died on 17 August 1349; born on *c.* 1 August 1304, he was 43 when his daughter was born and had recently turned 45 when he died. The widowed Hillaria married a second husband, Humphrey Swynnerton, and died in August 1372. Alice Bromley married John Frodesham in or before October 1362 when she was 15, and inherited from her father a wood called *Womworthyn* and a park called *Wilotebruggepark* in Ashley, a few miles from Eccleshall. Other people from the same area of Staffordshire who survived the Black Death and were still alive in the 1360s included Katherine Stretton, who was about the same age as Alice Bromley, Roger Pycheford, who was born in about 1312, Geoffrey Conegreve and his wife Agnes, Thomas Seyncler, born in about 1320, and Adam Cok, born in about 1309. In 1347, Adam Cok's daughter Juliana took her vows in Brewode Priory, a house of Benedictine nuns called *Blakladys* or 'Black Ladies' to distinguish it from a nearby priory called 'White Ladies'.[9]

Simon Ruggeleye was appointed sheriff of Staffordshire and Shropshire and constable of Shrewsbury Castle in 1336. He owned a house in Rugeley and rented a fishpond near Stafford called *Kyngespole* (King's Pool) 'by service of holding the king's currycomb on his first mounting his palfrey, every time of his coming to the town of Stafford'. Simon died on 9 August 1349. Unaware of Simon's death, Edward III appointed him and two other men on 31 August to seize goods belonging to a man in Staffordshire who owed the king a massive debt. Simon's son Humphrey, who was about 14 in 1349, was studying at Oxford, and if he survived the plague probably pursued a clerical career. The King's Pool was later held by the earls of Stafford (Ralph Stafford, the first earl, was born in 1301 and died in 1372).[10] William Trumwyn of Cannock died on 27 September 1349. His widow Alice was still alive in the summer of 1350, and their son William Trumwyn the younger, born in late September 1330, died in November 1361 leaving a 7-year-old daughter called Elizabeth and an 18-week-old son called John.[11]

In Glenfield near Leicester, the pestilence took a heavy toll on the Glenfeld family. Nicholas Glenfeld died on 11 June 1349, his father John died on *c.* 25 July 1349 and his son John the younger died on 6 October 1349. John the younger was 16 when he died, and his brother Baldwin, born sometime between July and November 1344, was barely 5 years old when he lost his brother, father and grandfather. Baldwin Glenfeld was alive in 1370 and dead by 1387.[12] Robert Poutrel of Prestwold near Loughborough in Leicestershire died on 12 June 1349. His three sisters, Maud Gotham, born *c.* Christmas 1328, Joan Prestwold, born *c.* 1 November 1330 and Cecily Poutrel, born *c.* 12 March 1332, survived and were all alive decades later.[13]

Gerard Seckyndon, step-grandfather of Elizabeth Garthorp of Wiverton in Nottinghamshire (see Chapter 11 above), came from Seckington in Warwickshire. Robert Burdet was born in Seckington on 26 October 1345 and survived the plague as a child, though his father, Robert Burdet the elder, did not; he died on 28 June 1349. At Robert the son's proof of age in November 1366, John Asshebrok recalled how Robert Burdet the father sent John as a messenger to his friends and well-wishers in Wiltshire, Staffordshire, Northamptonshire and Leicestershire in October 1345 to inform them of his son's birth and to express his joy at having a son. Henry Russell, born in *c.* 1308, remembered Robert Burdet the son's date of birth because his own (unnamed) father had been a tax collector in 1345, and when he went to Robert the father's house at the time that Robert the son was born, the father 'threatened [him] in life and limb so that he dared not approach his

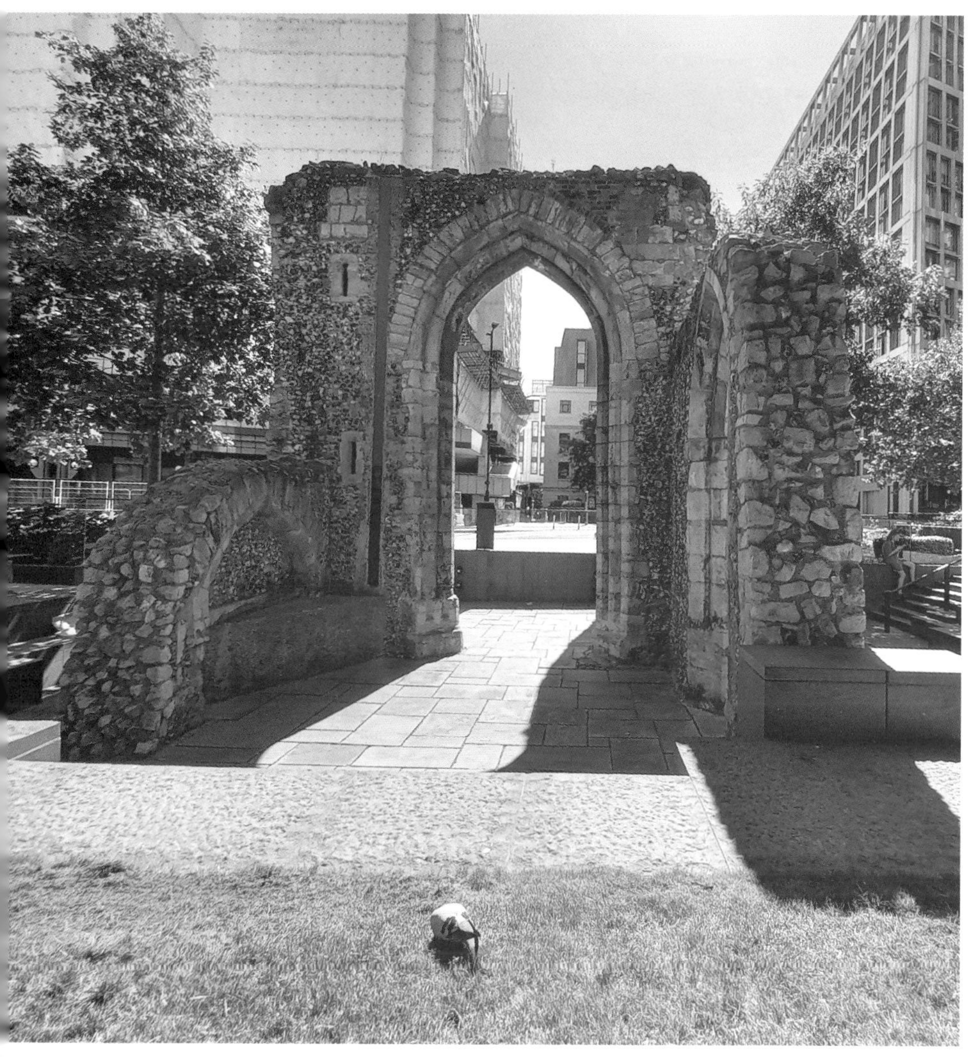

he remains of Elsyng Spital in the EC2 postal district of London, founded in 1330 by William Elsyng or lsing, who died between late March and early May 1349. His son Robert and daughter-in-law Alianore ed at almost the same time, and their son Thomas Elsing (b. 1346/47) survived all the pandemics of the lack Death and lived until 1431. (*It's No Game on Flickr*)

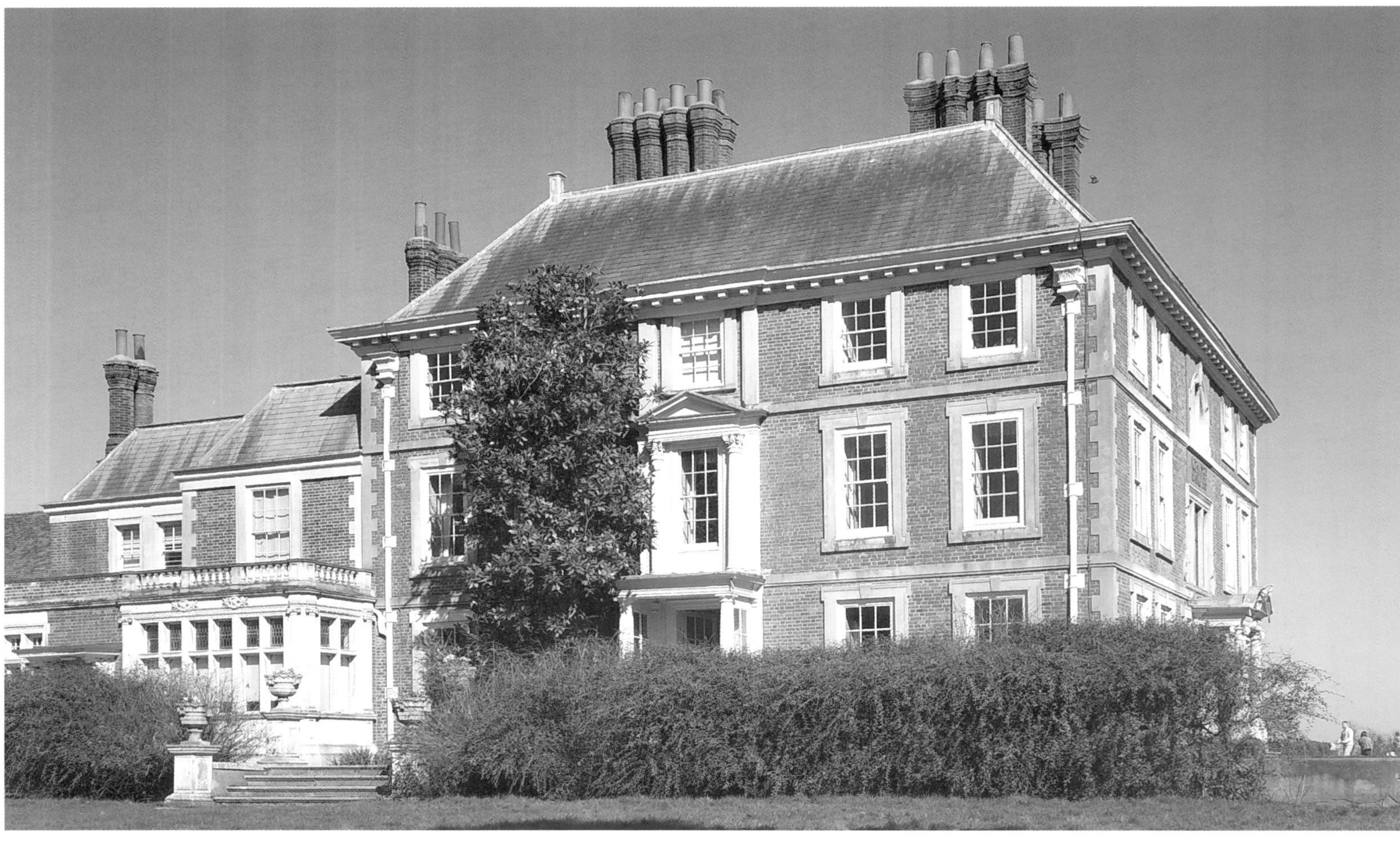

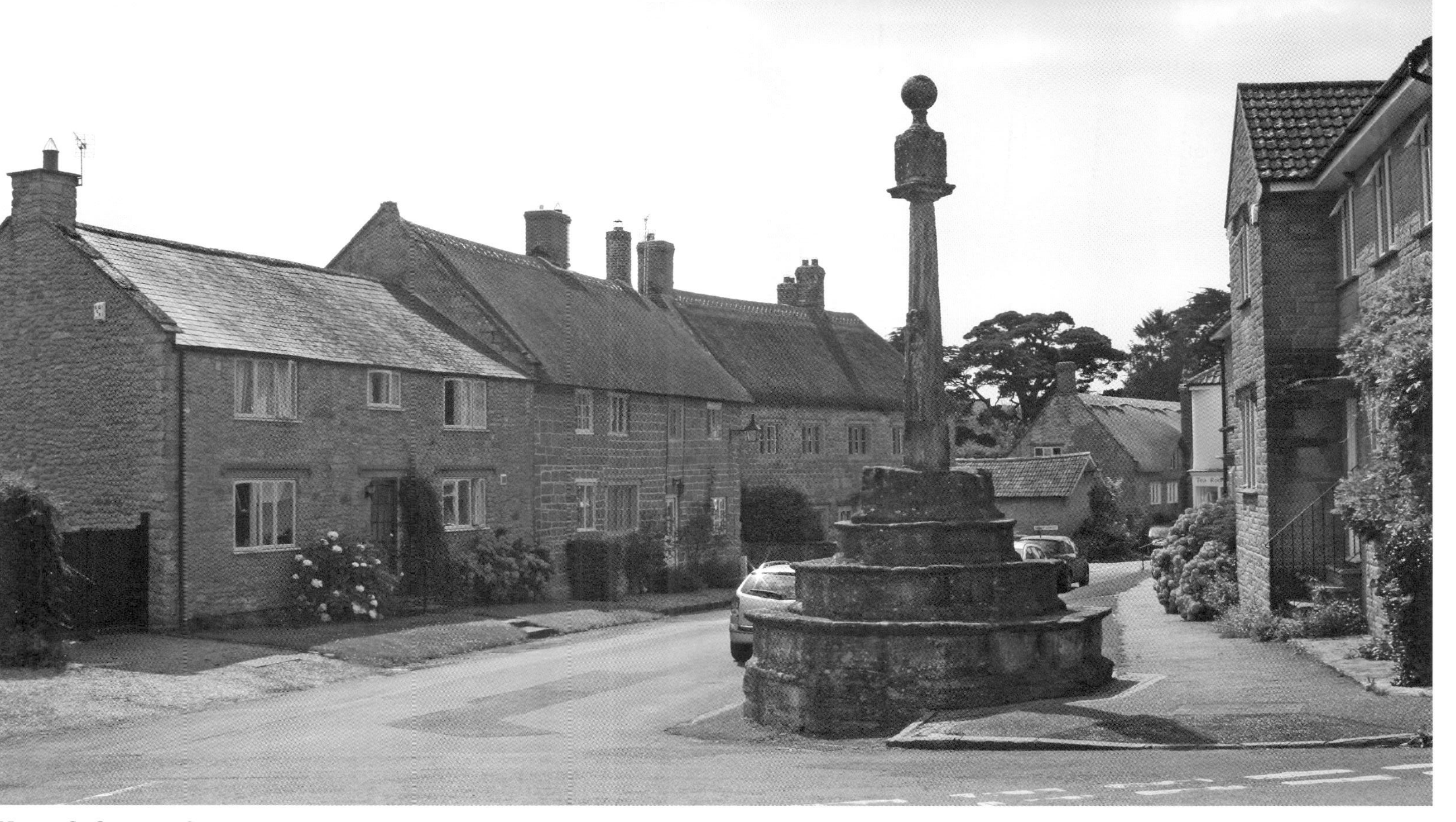

Hinton St George in Somerset, where John Warre died on 9 May 1349, just under two years after his son Richard was born in the village. Richard was still alive in the late 1360s. (*Nick Chipchase, Wikimedia Commons*)

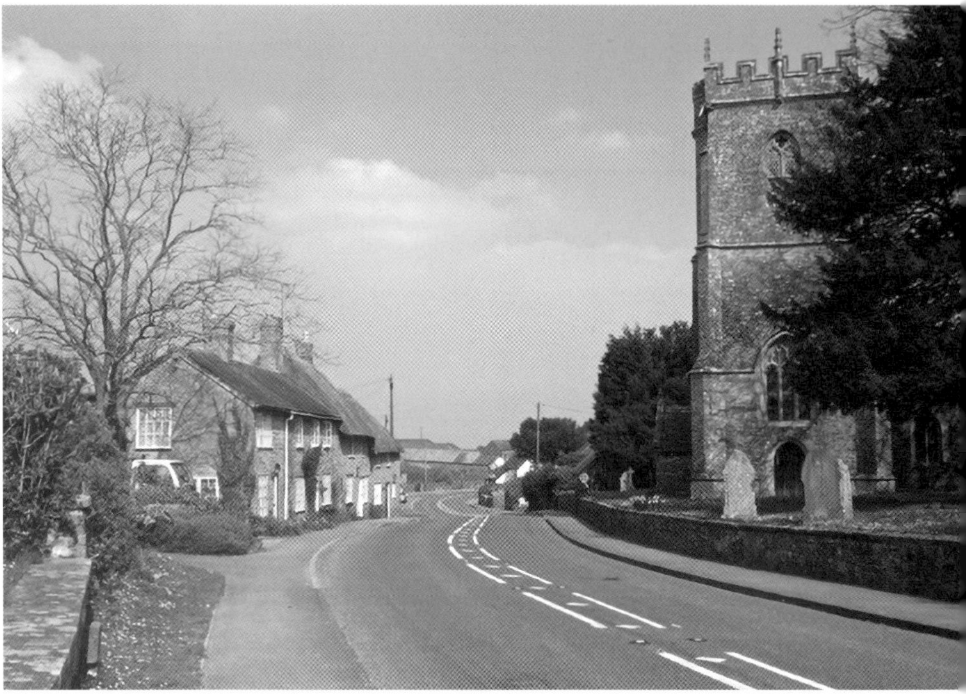

The Dorset village of Bishop's Caundle, where Thomas Keynes was born in July 1327. He proved that h
was now 21 in Sherborne in early October 1348, several months after the Black Death arrived in Melcomb
twenty-five miles away. (*Mike Searle, Wikimedia Commons*)

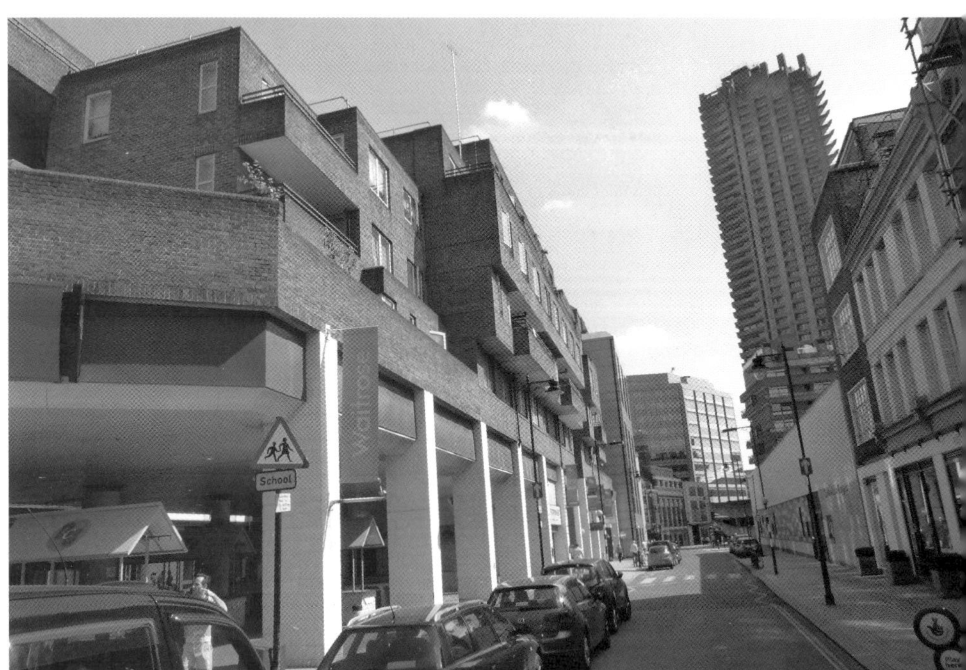

Whitecross Street, London EC1. Eight members of the Stokwell family of Whitecross Street died
1349, with just one survivor, 7-year-old Agnes. Having lost all her family, Agnes was placed in the care
her late father's apprentice. (*Gordon Joly, Flickr*)

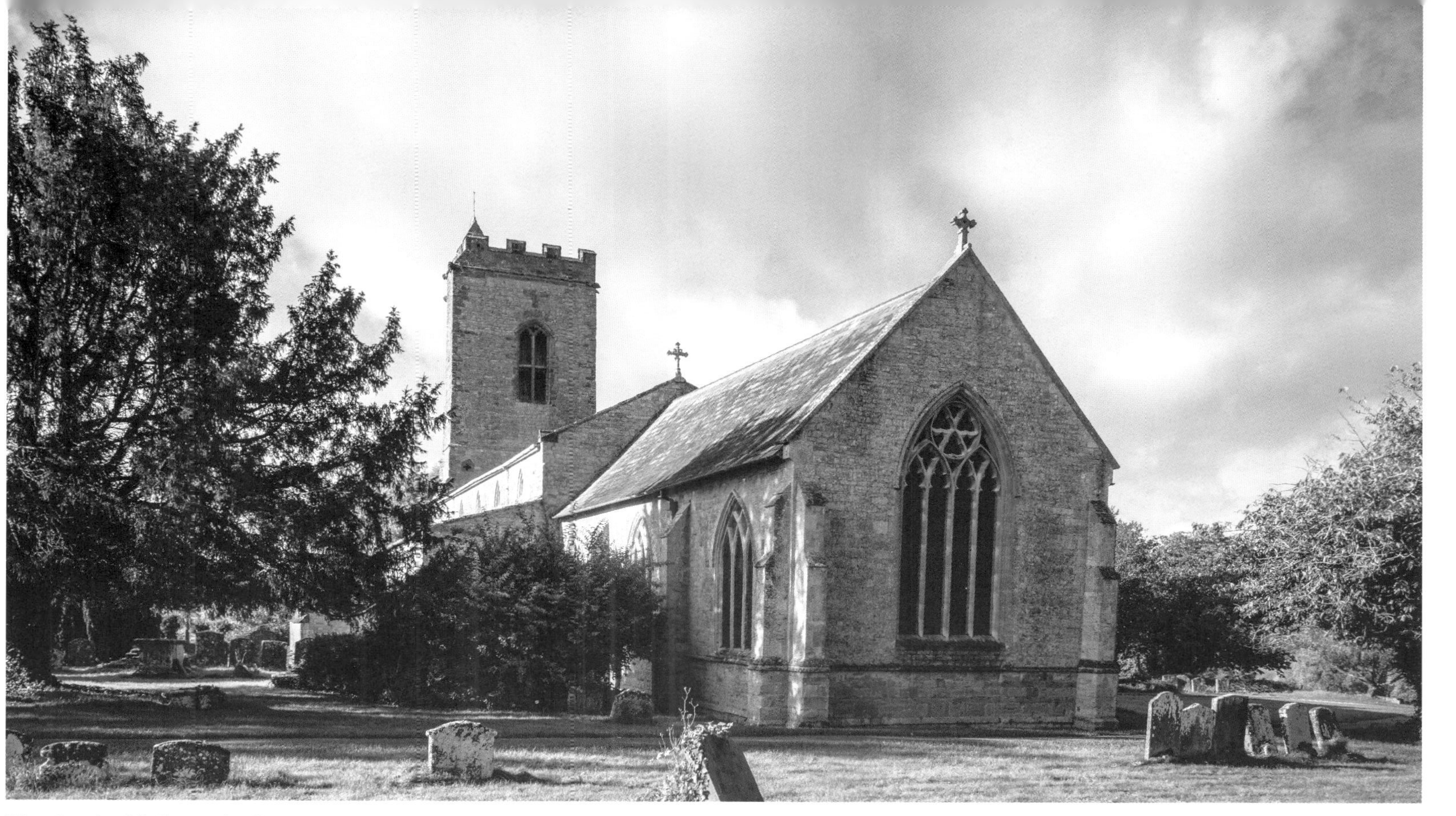

The church of St James the Great, Paulerspury, near Towcester in Northamptonshire. Sir Laurence Pavely (25 July 1327–7 June 1349) was buried here, and probably his brothers Roger and William, who also died in 1349, were as well. Only the fourth brother, John Pavely (b. 1333), survived. (*London Road, Flickr*)

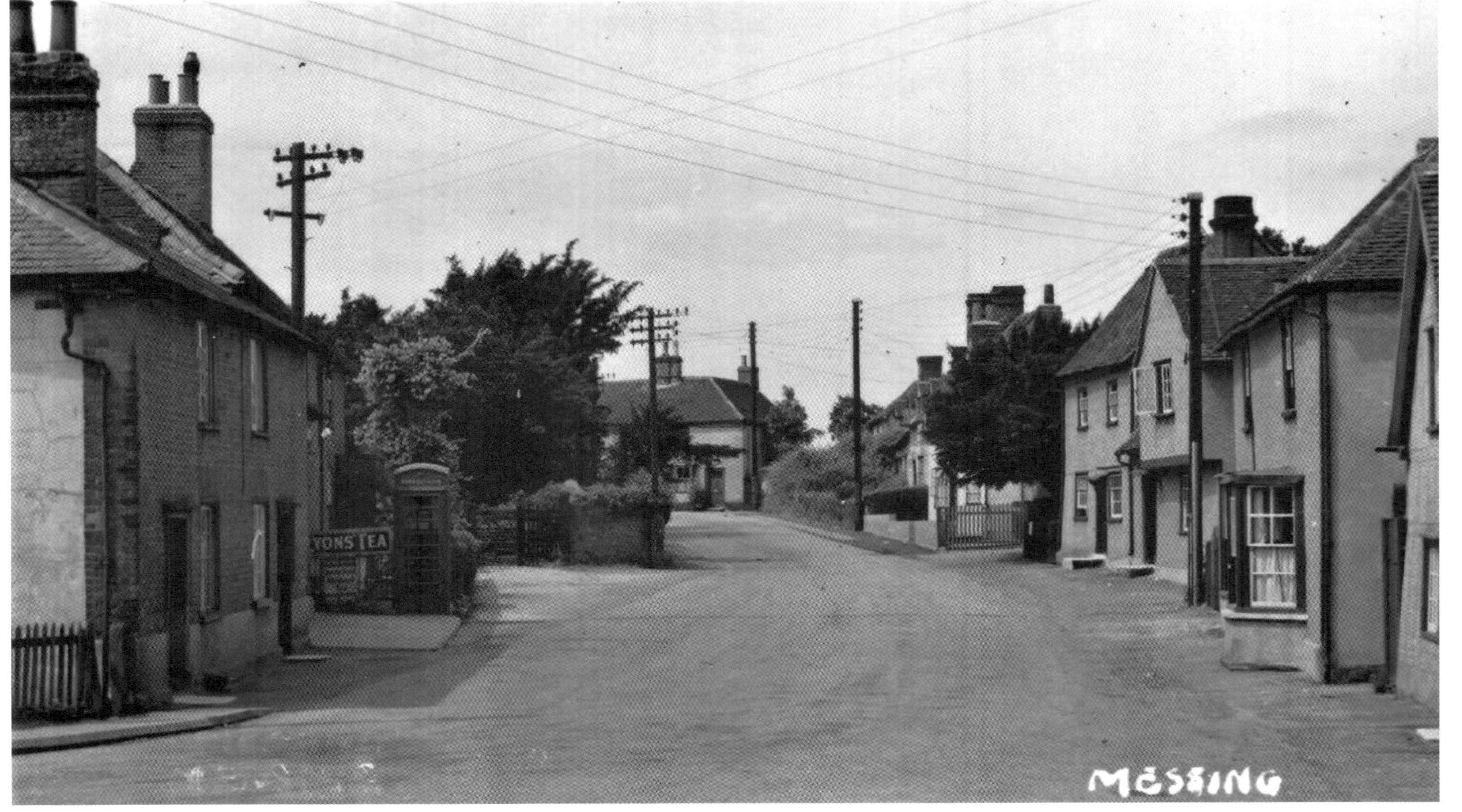

Messing, nine miles from Colchester in Essex, home of the Baynard family. At least four members of the family died during the fourth pandemic of 1375, a quarter of

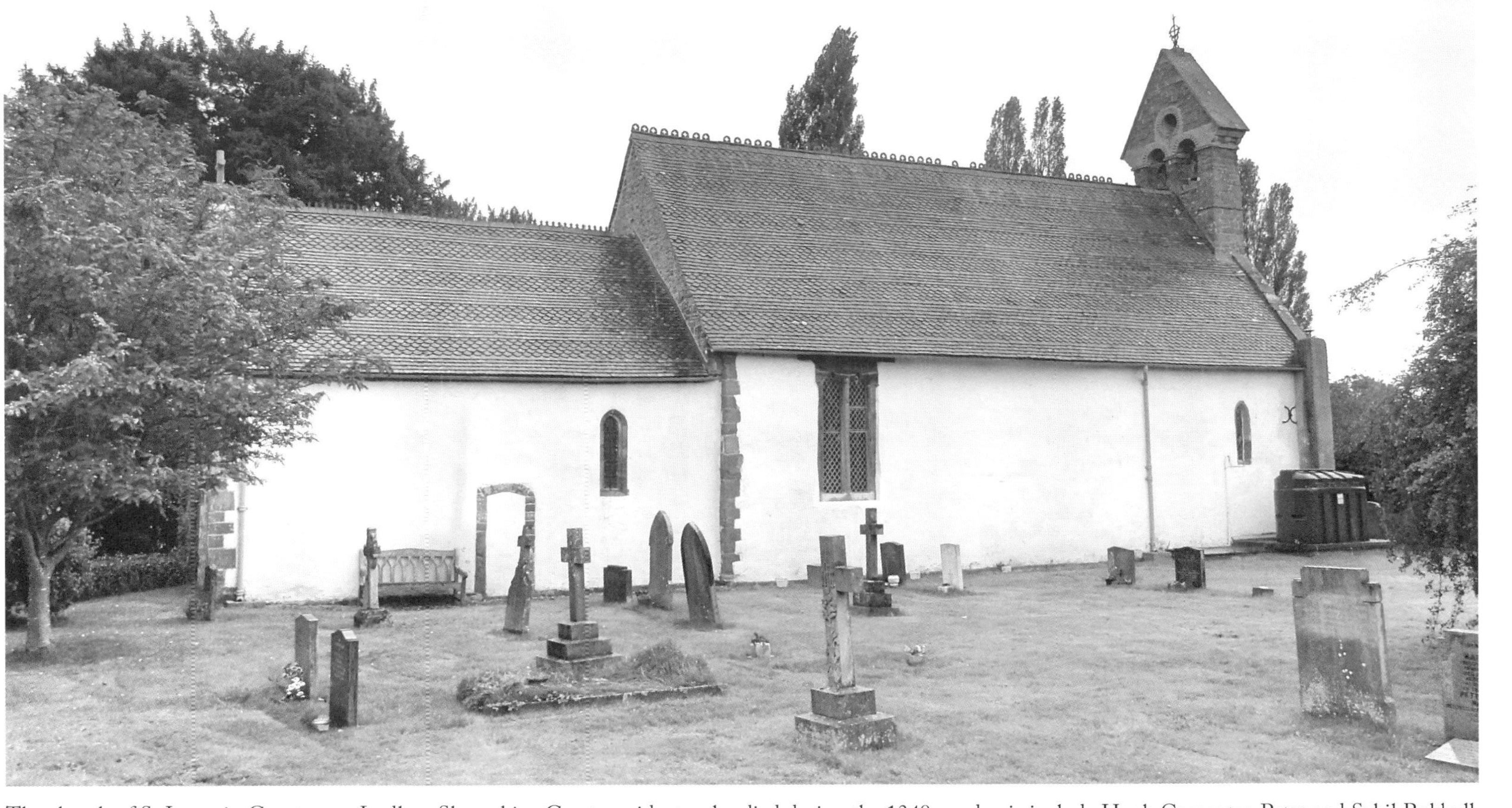

The church of St James in Greete near Ludlow, Shropshire. Greete residents who died during the 1349 pandemic include Hugh Carpenter, Peter and Sybil Rokhull, William Stoke and Agnes Halughton. Hugh Carpenter's daughters Margery, Agnes and Isabel might have died in the second pandemic of 1361, though their youngest sister Alice (b. September 1341) survived both. (*Philip Pankhurst, Wikimedia Commons*)

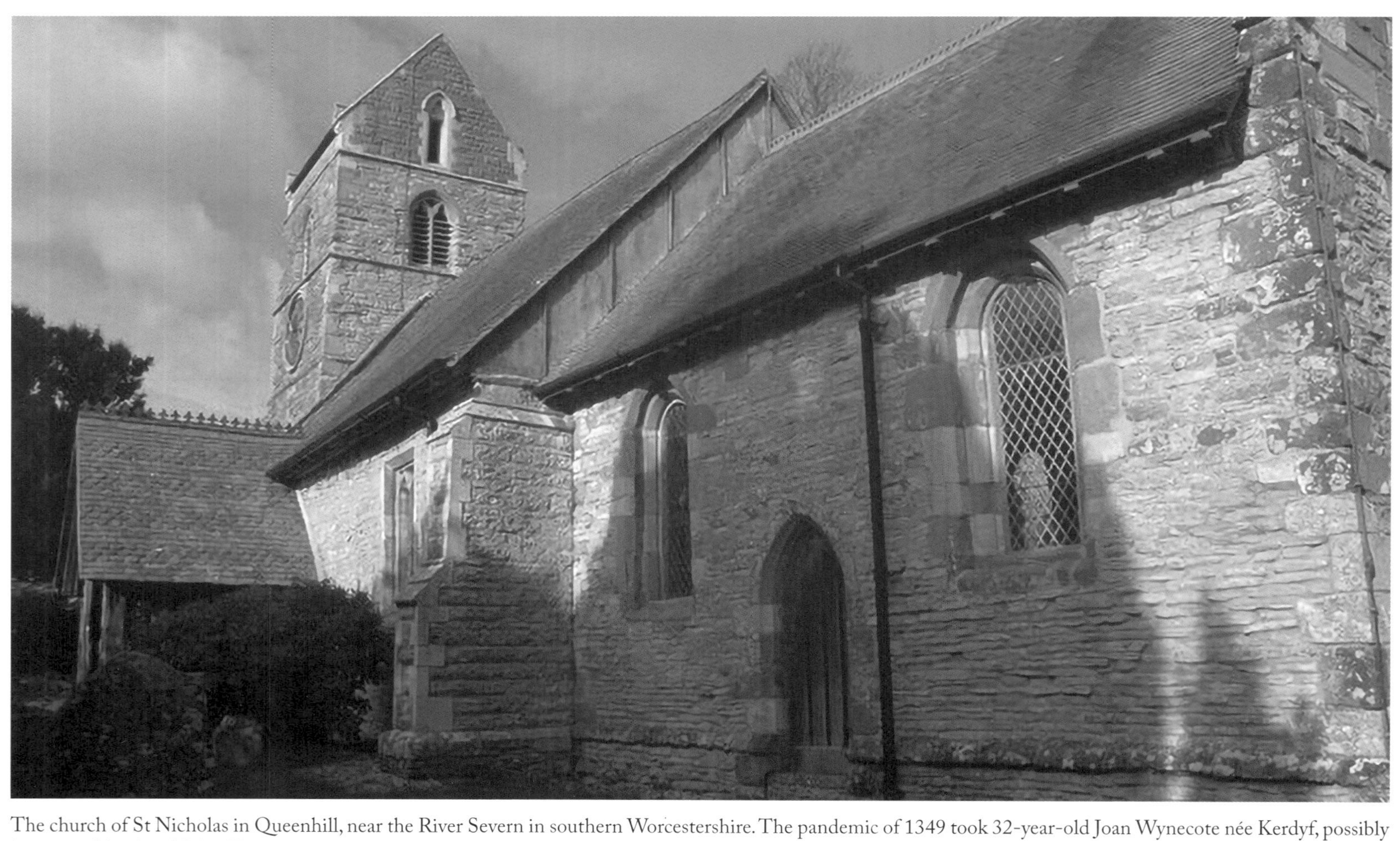

The church of St Nicholas in Queenhill, near the River Severn in southern Worcestershire. The pandemic of 1349 took 32-year-old Joan Wynecote née Kerdyf, possibly

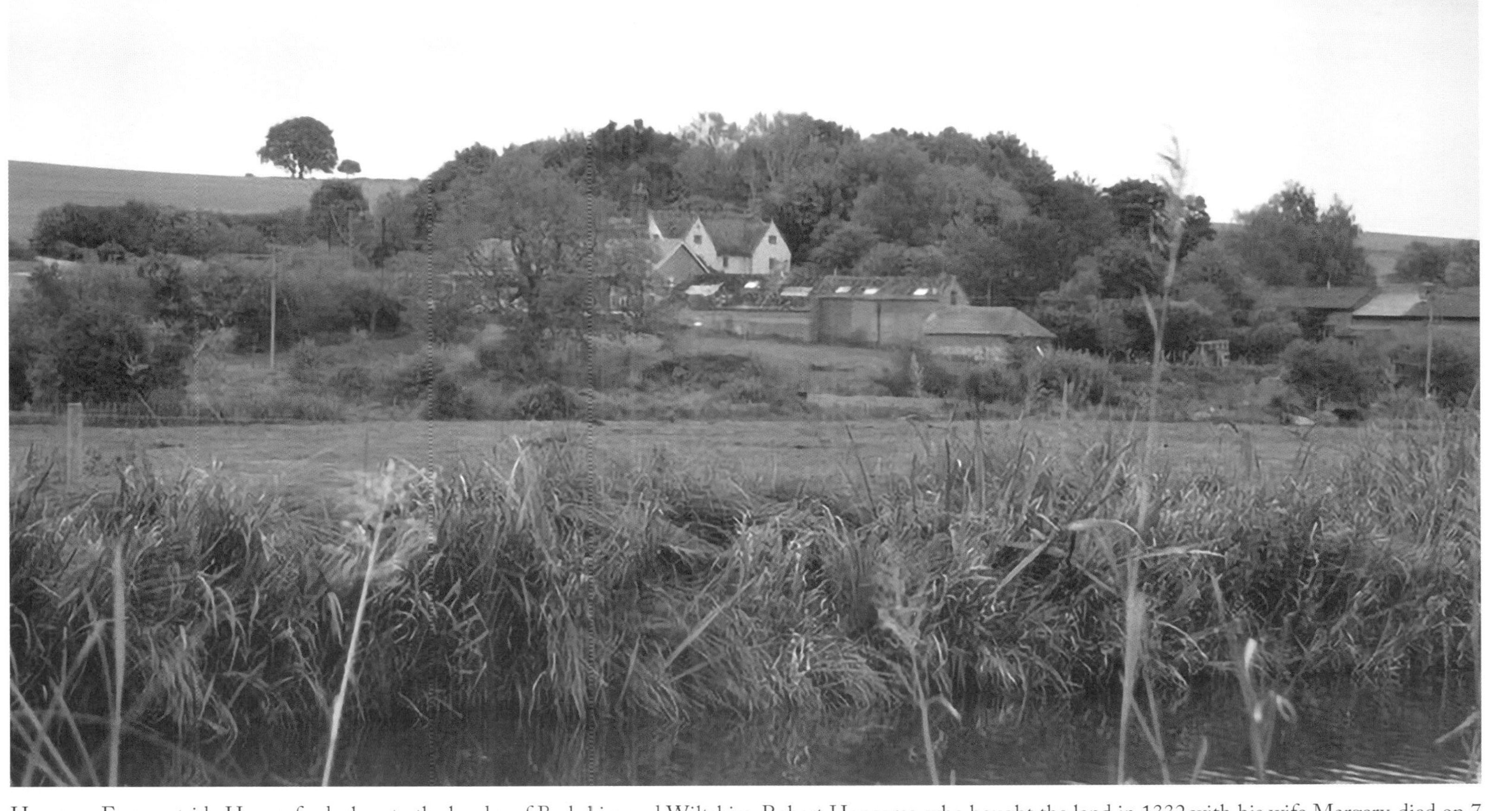

Hopgrass Farm outside Hungerford, close to the border of Berkshire and Wiltshire. Robert Hopegras, who bought the land in 1332 with his wife Margery, died on 7 June 1349, and their 24-year-old son Richard died on 13 June 1349. Richard's son William Hopegras, about 6 in 1349, died between September 1417 and June 1423. (*N. Chadwick, Geograph*)

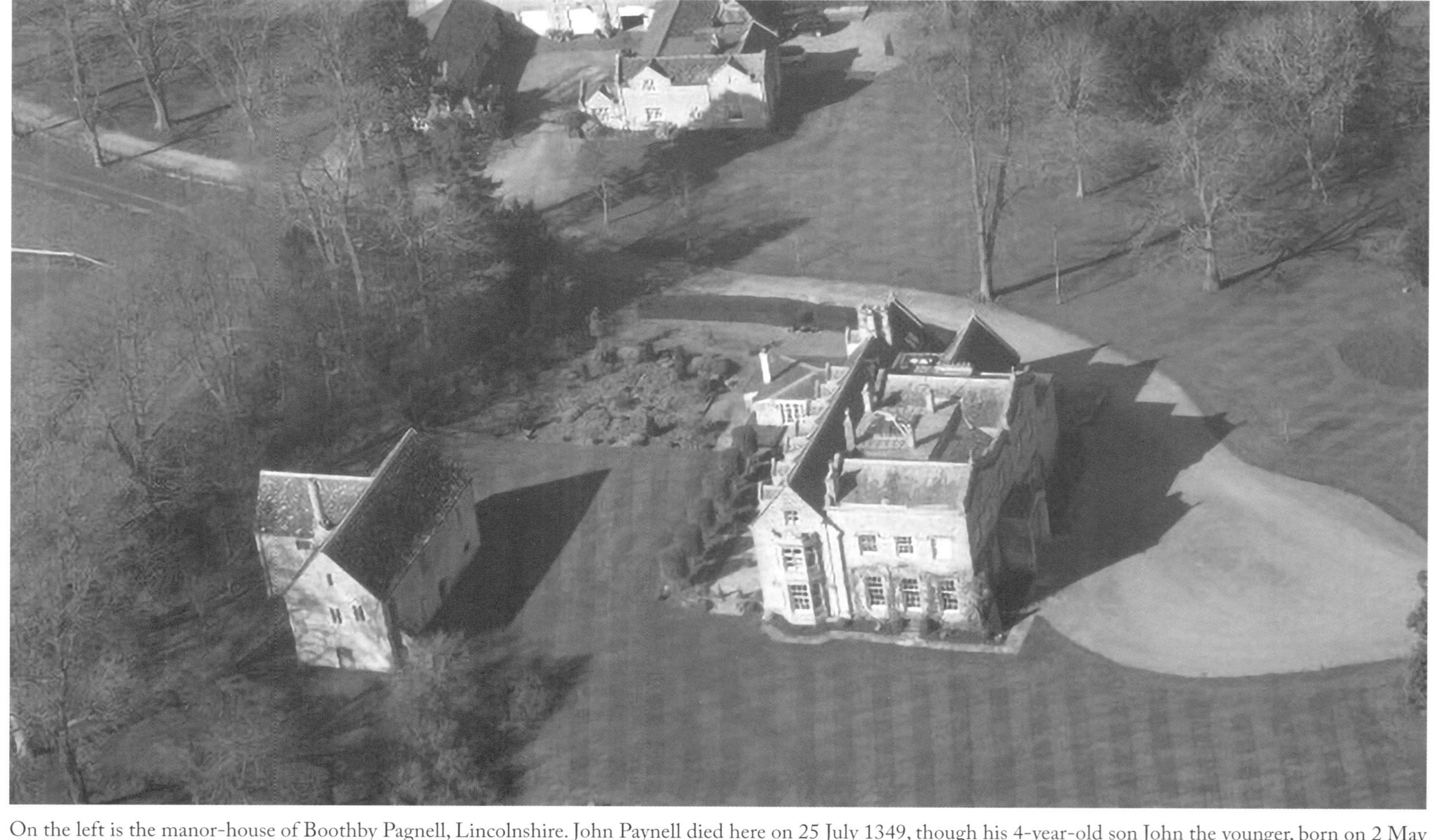

On the left is the manor-house of Boothby Pagnell, Lincolnshire. John Paynell died here on 25 July 1349, though his 4-year-old son John the younger, born on 2 May 1345 … [illegible]

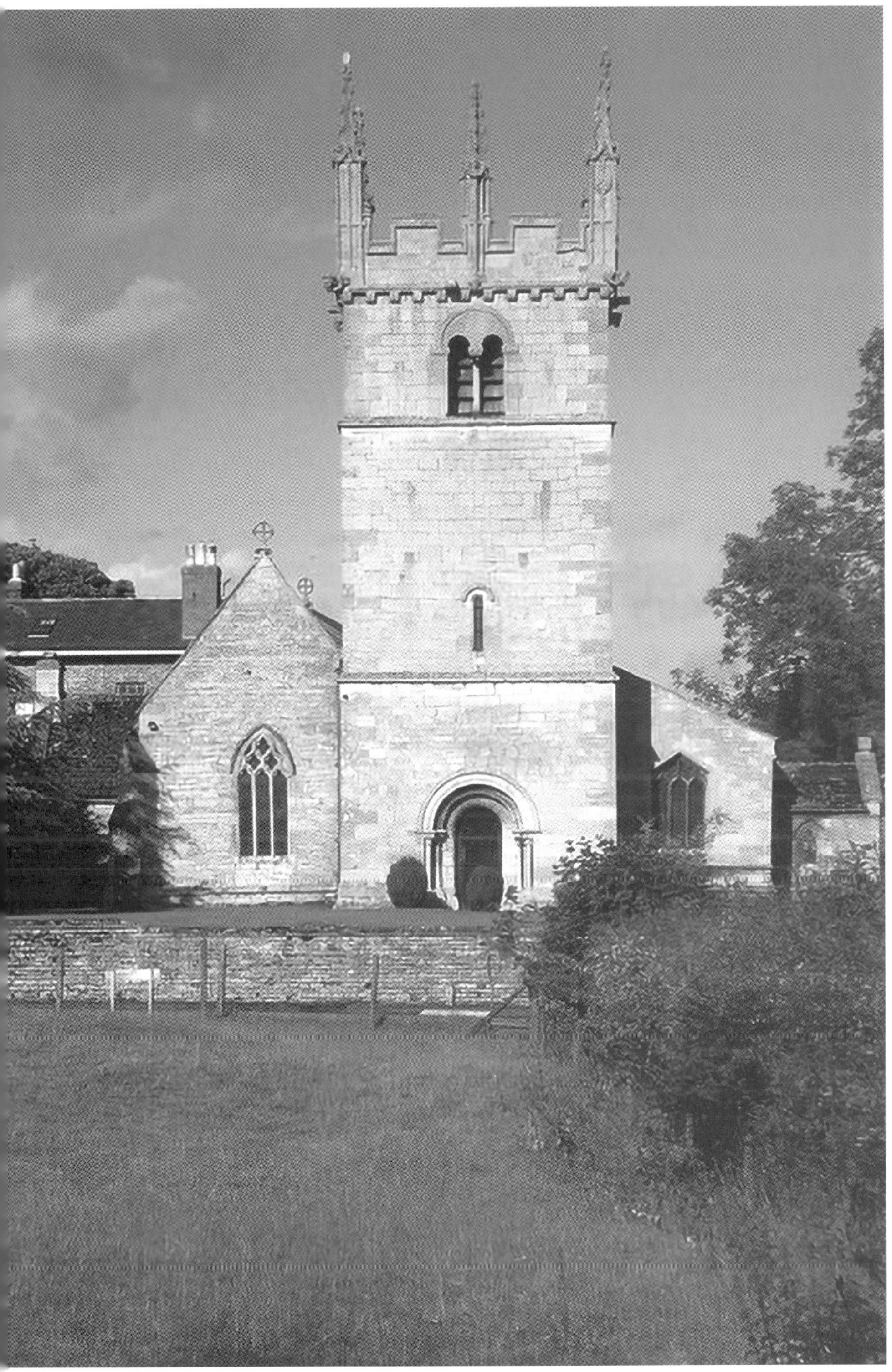

St Andrew's church in Boothby Pagnell, where John Paynell the younger was baptised by the local parson, Richard Pynzon, on 2 May 1345. Edmund Kyrnell, baptised here on 3 May 1345, and his older brother William, also lived through the first pandemic. (*Stefan Czapski, Geograph*)

PENSHURST PLACE
PRIVATE ENTRANCE
PUBLIC ENTRANCE TO
HOUSE AND GROUNDS
THROUGH VILLAGE

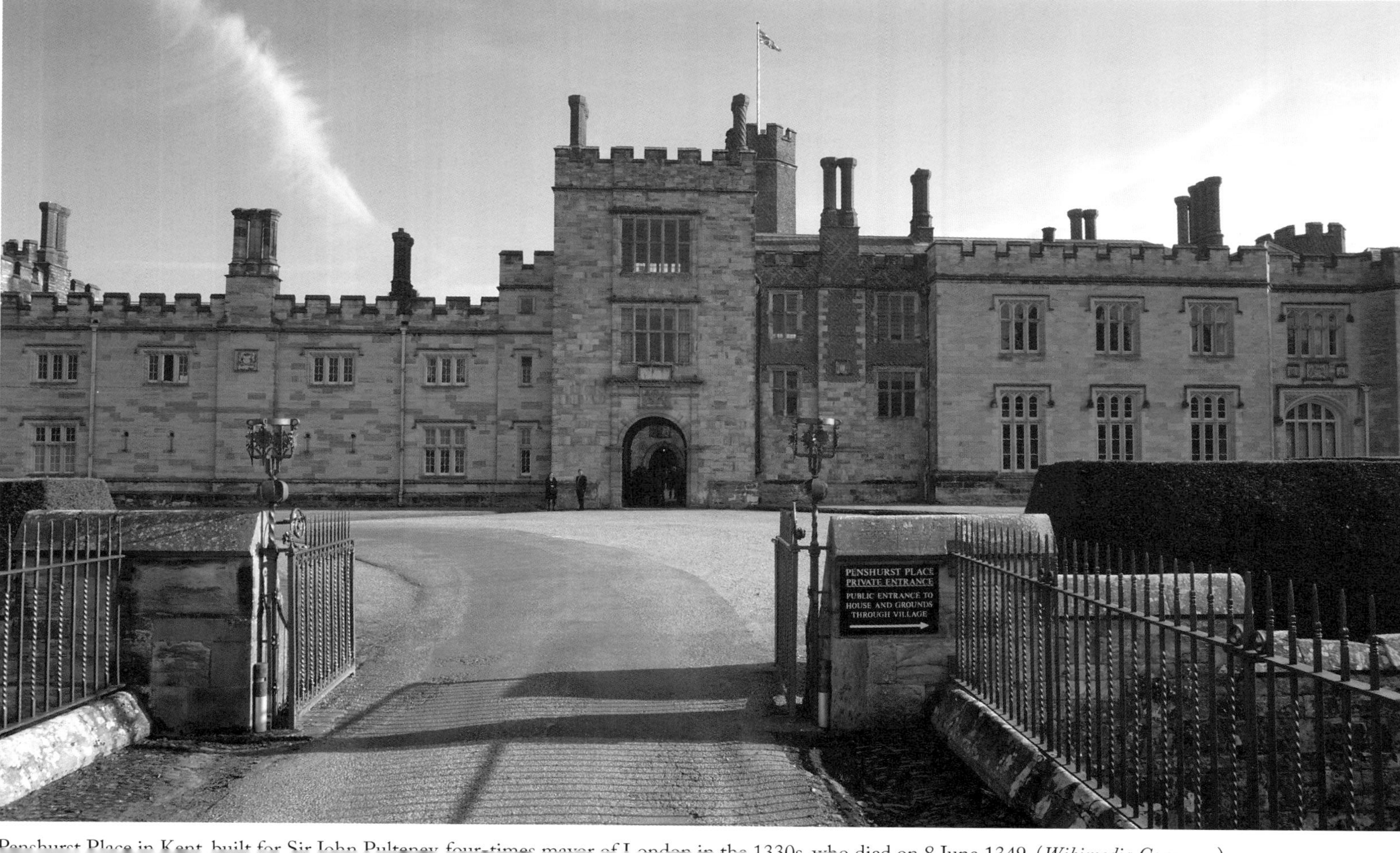

Penshurst Place in Kent, built for Sir John Pulteney, four-times mayor of London in the 1330s, who died on 8 June 1349. (*Wikimedia Commons*)

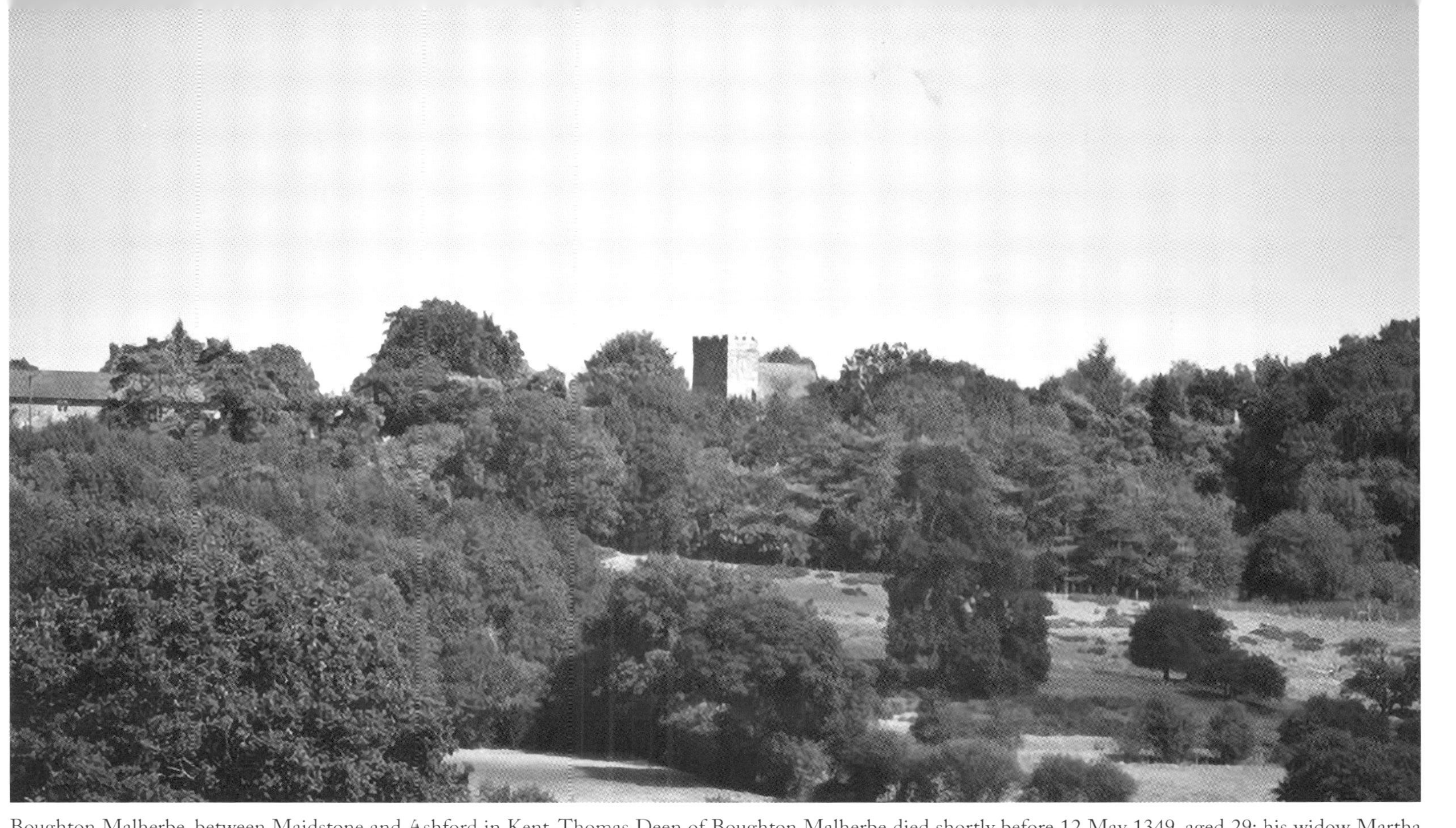

Boughton Malherbe, between Maidstone and Ashford in Kent. Thomas Deen of Boughton Malherbe died shortly before 12 May 1349, aged 29; his widow Martha died before 7 June 1349; and all four of their daughters, aged 5, 4, 2 and 1, were dead by 30 June 1349. (*N. Chadwick, Geograph*)

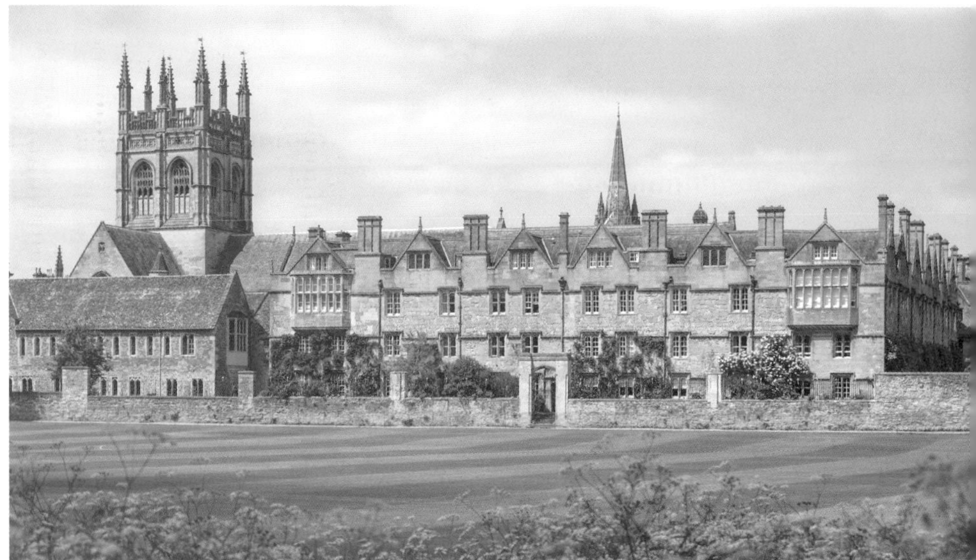

Merton College at the University of Oxford. In the 1330s and 1340s, it was a centre of advanced mathematica and logical thought thanks to a group of men known as the Oxford Calculators. They included Thoma Bradwardine, briefly archbishop of Canterbury, and John Dumbleton, who both died of plague in 134 (*Jonas Magnus Lystad, Wikimedia Commons*)

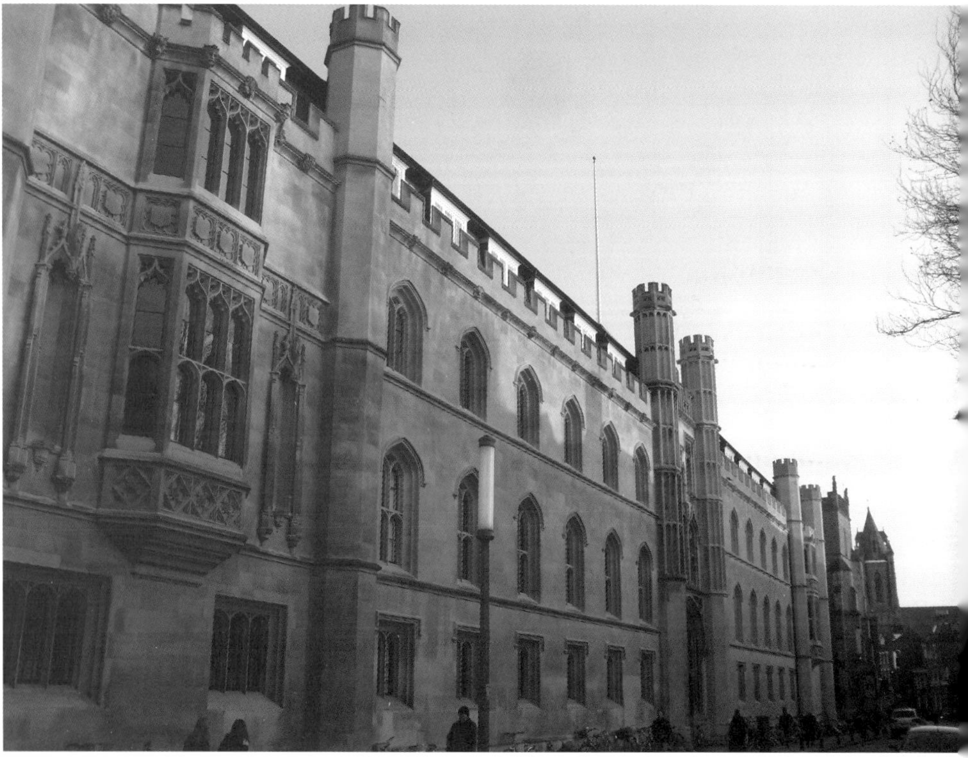

Corpus Christi College at the University of Cambridge, founded in 1352 by some of the townspeople o Cambridge who had recently survived the Black Death. (*McAnt, Wikimedia Commons*)

he site of Hampole Priory near Doncaster in Yorkshire, where the hermit and mystic Richard Rolle died n 30 September 1349. (*John Armagh, Wikimedia Commons*)

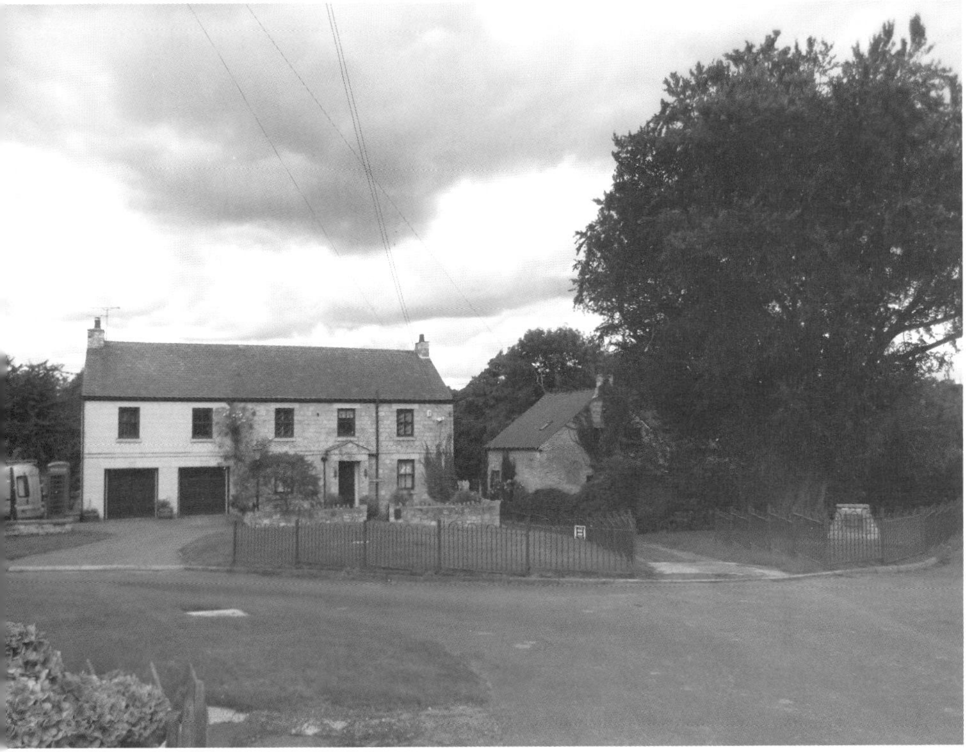

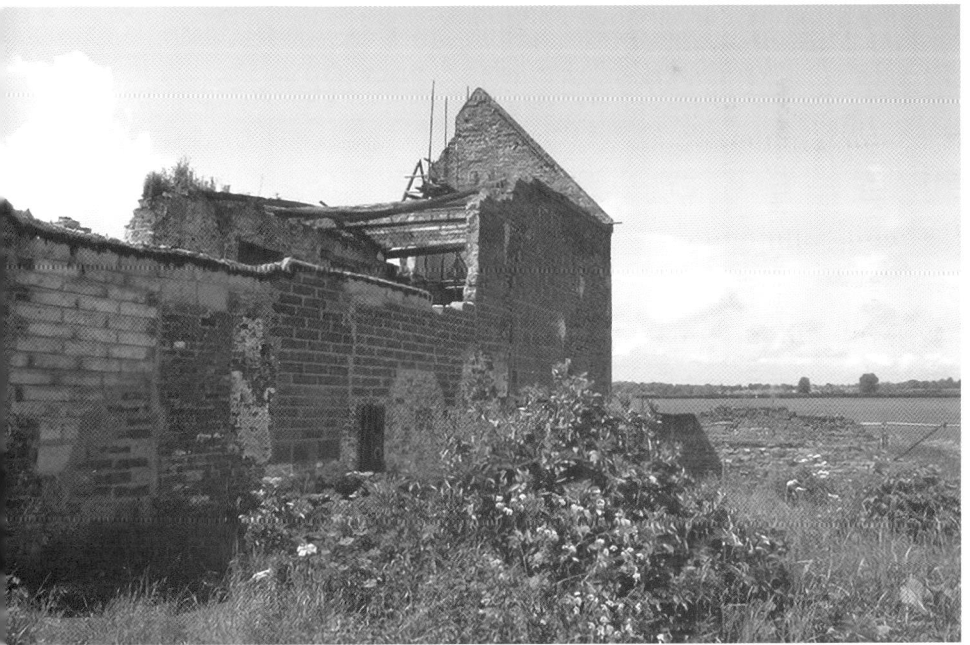

he remains of Haltemprice Priory Farm near Hull in Yorkshire. The priory was founded by Thomas, ord Wake, who died on 30 May 1349. His sister and heir Margaret, countess of Kent, died just four ıonths later. (*Paul Glazzard, Geograph*)

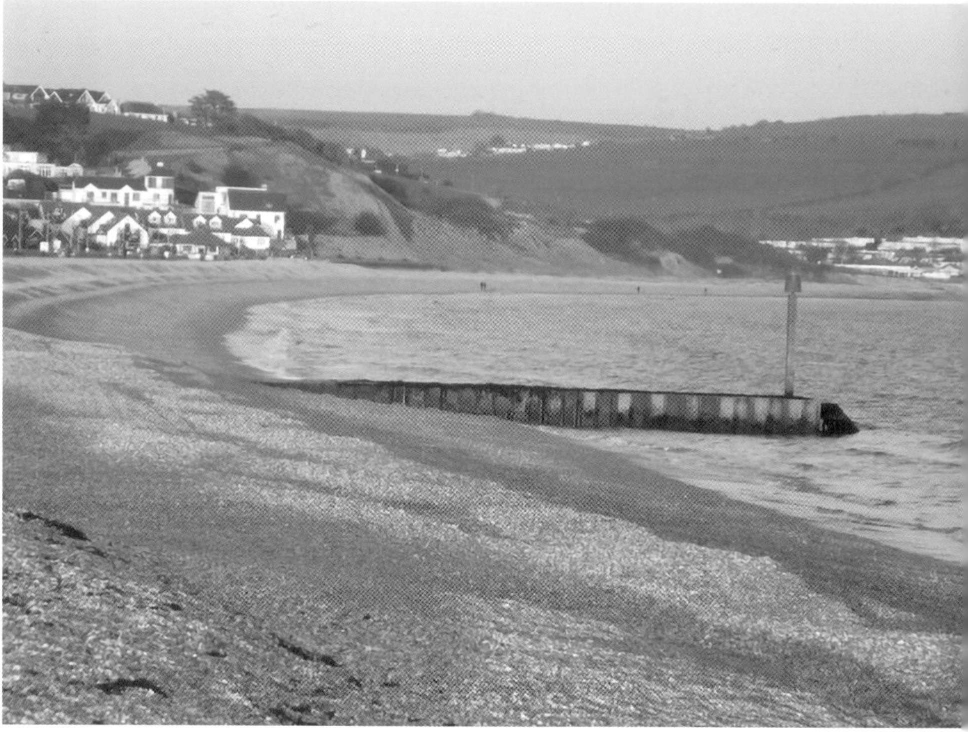

The beach of Melcombe in Dorset, now called Melcombe Regis and part of Weymouth. Several fourteenth century chroniclers state that the Black Death arrived in Melcombe from the Continent in the summe of 1348. (*Colin Smith, Geograph*)

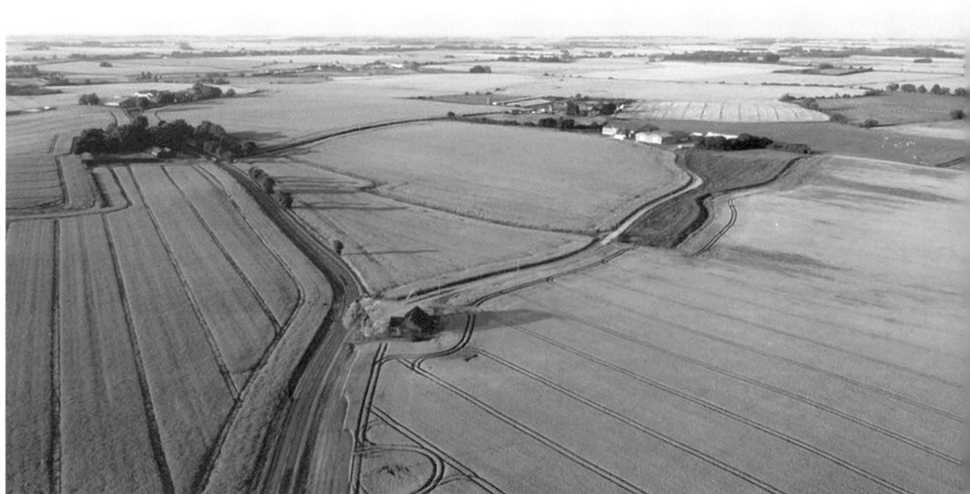

Part of the flat, low-lying Holderness peninsula near Hull, Yorkshire. This part of England suffered terribly high death rate between July and September 1349. (*Andy Beecroft, Geograph*)

house'. Gerard Burdet of Seckington, presumably a relative, died on 9 July 1349, leaving a 3-year-old son, John.[14]

Two other Warwickshire victims were Roger atte Hall of Alcester, who was born on 12 March 1332 and was 17 when he died in the summer of 1349, and Elizabeth Botreaux also of Alcester, who died on 20 July 1349. Elizabeth's son Walter was born on the same day as Roger atte Hall, and survived. In the Warwickshire village of Wappenbury, south of Coventry, it was said in October 1350 that eight homes and eighty acres of land were untenanted because of the pestilence.[15] And John Loges from Sowe in Warwickshire – this presumably means Walsgrave on the River Sowe, close to Coventry – died on 10 August 1349.[16] He was born around 1311/13 as the son of Nicholas Warrewyk and Elizabeth Loges, so was about 36 or 38 when he died, and used his mother's family name. His mother Elizabeth, born in 1293, died in 1315 when her son was little, and her mother Elizabeth the elder, widow of Richard Loges (d. 1300), married again twice before she died in 1337.[17] In *c.* 1303, Elizabeth the elder – the grandmother of John Loges who died in 1349 – was abducted in Rodbaston, Staffordshire, by Adam Staneye, whom she later married, willingly or not. The couple were sued for 'causing waste and destruction in the woods' that were part of Elizabeth's daughter Elizabeth Loges' inheritance. Adam Staneye was still alive in March 1319, but by July 1321 Elizabeth was married to her third husband, John Saundrestede, who outlived his step-grandson John Loges and died in 1353.[18]

The Loges/Warrewyk/Peyto Family of Warwickshire

Richard Loges (1265–1300) m. Elizabeth (d. 1337) who m. 2)Adam Staneye (d. *c.* 1320) and m.3) John Saundrestede (d. 1353)

|

Elizabeth Loges (1293–1315) m. Nicholas Warrewyk

|

John Loges (*c.* 1311/13–49) m. Margaret (d. before 1349)

|

John (alive 1344, d. before 1349)
Eleanor (*c.* 1332/33–before 1396) m. John Peyto (d. 1396)

|

William Peyto (d. 1407)

John Loges married a woman called Margaret, and they had two children. Their son John the younger was alive in 1344 and was married to Isabella, but he must have died before John (as did Margaret).[19] Their only other child was Eleanor, who was born in 1332 or 1333 and was old enough to know her great-grandmother Elizabeth (d. 1337). At the time of the Black Death, Eleanor was already married to John Peyto, who was probably about the same age as she, and they both lived through the pandemic. In May 1352, Eleanor Loges' father-in-law William Peyto witnessed a grant alongside her step-great-grandfather John Saundrestede.[20] The date of Eleanor's death is not recorded, though she was already dead when her husband John Peyto died in February 1396. They had a son, named William after his paternal grandfather.[21]

Chapter 14

Essex and Kent

John Sayer of Latchingdon in Essex, who was at the start of his 30s, died on 24 May 1349, and his younger brother Hugh Sayer died on 18 June. John left two very young sons: Richard, probably born in the first few months of 1346, and John, born in Copford, Essex on 1 November 1347. Richard Sayer survived the first pandemic of 1348/49 but died around Christmas in 1361, aged 15, during the second pandemic. His younger brother John proved his age in Colchester in late 1368. One of the jurors, Robert atte Holte, remembered John's birth in November 1347 because shortly afterwards he fell over some casks on a ship and broke his arm. Richard Noth remembered because about a month before John was born, he took his horse on the Fambridge ferry (*Fambreggeferye*). A sudden storm blew up, and the panicked horse leapt from the ferry into the sea, though thankfully survived. Two other jurors related alarming stories as their reasons for remembering John Sayer's birth. Stephen Richer, who was 22 in 1347, stated that, around the time that John was born, Stephen's father killed his mother, and John Sumpter said that a few weeks before John Sayer's birth, he had gone out on his cart in autumn and 'killed John his servant with a [pitch]fork'. He failed to explain the motive for this murder, and as he was still only 37 when he related the story at John Sayer's proof of age in late 1368, he must only have been 16 when it occurred.[1]

Another Essex victim of the plague was William Cosyn of Stansted Mountfitchet, who died on 20 April 1349 when his son John, born *c.* 1344, was 4 or 5.[2] John Cosyn was still alive in 1390, and a few miles from Stansted Mountfitchet, the Walden family also survived the pandemic. Andrew Walden was born on 20 November 1311 in Saffron Walden (then called 'Chepingwaleden' or Chipping Walden) and named after his godfather Andrew Thunderley, and his son Thomas Walden was born in Magdalen Laver (then called 'Maudeleynlavar' or 'Laufar Magdeleyne') on 31 October 1345. Andrew died on 8 August 1352, and his wife Joan, Thomas's mother, on 23 August 1361. They also had a daughter named Alice, whose date of birth is not known. Thomas Walden died on 9 May 1420 at the age of 74, leaving no children; his heir was his sister Alice's son Thomas Bataille (d. 1439).[3] Edmund Amory of Little Maldon in Essex died on 30 May 1349, and must still have been a young man; his brother John was born on 6 November 1331.[4]

The Coggeshale, Baynard and Welle families of Essex suffered in two outbreaks of the Black Death. Sir John Coggeshale – his family name means the Essex village of Coggeshall – was born in 1301 and served four terms as sheriff of Essex between 1334 and 1354.[5] He had a son Henry, born in *c.* 1331, and a daughter Isabel, who must have been a few years older than her brother, as she married John Baynard and gave birth to their son Thomas Baynard on 14 September 1337 (and can therefore hardly have been born later than 1322). Thomas Baynard was born in the home of his maternal grandfather, the sheriff John Coggeshale, in Codham in the parish of Wethersfield.[6] His uncle Henry Coggeshale married a woman named Joan Welle, who confusingly was only two years older than Thomas. The only child of William and Agnes Welle, Joan was born on 8 September 1335 in Great Sampford, six miles from the Coggeshale family home near Wethersfield, and twenty-five miles from the Baynards' home in the village of Messing.[7]

The Coggeshale and Baynard Families of Essex

Sir John Coggeshale, sheriff of Essex
(1301–61)

Isabel (d. 1375) m. John Baynard (d. 1349)	Henry Coggeshale (*c.* 1331–75) m. Joan Welle (1335–75)
Thomas Baynard (1337–75) m. Katherine (d. 1375?)	William (1358–1426) Thomas (I) Thomas (II) Other children
Richard (b. 1371) John Robert Thomas	

Isabel Coggeshale's mother-in-law Joan Baynard died on 20 September 1349, and Isabel's husband John Baynard on 4 November; Thomas Baynard was 12 when he lost his father and grandmother. William Welle, whose daughter Joan married Isabel's younger brother Henry Coggeshale, died on

13 April 1349, and as there is no mention of Joan's mother Agnes afterwards, she was either already dead or also a victim of the plague. Neighbours of the Baynards in Messing were the Belhous family, and little Thomas Belhous, born in the village on 14 February 1347, lived through the pestilence and died on 9 August 1374 leaving a 4-year-old daughter. Thomas's sister Isolde Belhous also survived.[8]

Isabel, her brother Henry, and their father all survived the Black Death, as did Isabel's son Thomas Baynard, who proved in 1359 that he had now come of age. Two years later, on 4 June 1361, his maternal grandfather John Coggeshale died at the age of 60. John's heir was his then 30-year-old son Henry, followed by Henry and Joan Welle's eldest son William Coggeshale, born on 20 July 1358 in his grandfather John's home in Codham, as his much older cousin Thomas Baynard had also been, two decades earlier. Henry Coggeshale and Joan Welle had other children too: an inquisition talks of the couple 'having many sons and daughters to maintain', and confusingly two of their younger sons both bore the name Thomas.[9] Henry's cousin Thomas Baynard married a woman called Katherine, and they had four sons born in the first half of the 1370s called Richard, John, Robert and Thomas.[10]

Joan Coggeshale née Welle died on 27 September 1375; her husband Henry Coggeshale died on 29 September 1375; Henry's cousin Thomas Baynard died on 8 October 1375; and Thomas's mother Isabel Baynard née Coggeshale died on 6 November 1375.[11] It seems almost impossible that four members of a family could die so closely together by mere chance, and is highly likely that they all fell victim to a virulently infectious disease, perhaps the fourth pandemic of the Black Death, in the mid-1370s. Katherine Baynard, Thomas's widow, was alive on 8 November 1375, two days after her mother-in-law Isabel died, then disappears from history. Their eldest son Richard, born *c.* February 1371, was alive on 22 October 1376 then also vanishes.[12] After 1375/76, the rather well-documented Baynard family become almost impossible to find on record, and it seems that neither Richard Baynard nor any of his three brothers lived into adulthood. Their father's cousin William Coggeshale did survive: he was appointed sheriff of Essex in 1404 and died in March 1426 when he was 67.[13]

John atte Brok of White Roding in Essex died around Christmas 1348, leaving his son Thomas, born *c.* 7 July 1328, in possession of the house he owned there called *Maskelesbury*.[14] Beatrice Quenton also of White Roding died on 1 July 1349, and her daughter Alice, age not recorded, died only fifteen days later. William Quenton, Beatrice's husband and Alice's father, survived.[15] John Liston, son of John and Maud Liston, was born in the village of Liston in Essex, close to the Suffolk border, on 2 February 1336, 19 months before Thomas Baynard was born 15 miles away. John Liston the father died on 24 July 1349 in his late 30s, and his wife Maud died around the same time. John the son, 13 years old in 1349, survived the plague, as did his uncles, William and Thomas Liston, his father's brothers, and his uncle-in-law John Naylingherst, who married his father's sister Alice Liston in September 1336 and was one of the jurors who took part in Thomas Baynard's proof of age in Braintree in 1359. John Liston the son proved his age in August 1357, but did not have much longer to live: he died on military service in Normandy around 25 January 1359, shortly before his twenty-third birthday. He had not married and left no children, and his heir was his uncle William Liston.[16]

Another young Essex man who survived the plague was James Tracy, born in Stanford Rivers on 18 May 1327. John Couk from Navestock, three miles away, was staying with James's parents Thomas and Mabel when James was born, and 'heard the cries of the mother' as she gave birth to James. John Pikerel, who was about 37 in 1327 and was still alive at the end of the 1340s, was one of the villagers in church listening to Mass when 'the midwives came and announced the birth of the said James'. Thomas Tracy, James's father, died in early 1335, and James was placed in the wardship of Mabel FitzWarin, an attendant of Queen Philippa. He survived the Black Death but, like his rather younger contemporary John Liston, did not live past his 20s: James Tracy died in late October 1353.[17]

Thomas and Mary Fabel owned a house called Benfletes in Hatfield Peverel, Essex with 120 acres of land, 3 acres of meadow, 12 of pasture and 4 of wood. Thomas had a younger brother called William Fabel, who was a clerk, and they had an illegitimate half-brother too, son of their father and his lover Agnes Ultynge, who was known as both John Fabel and John Ultynge. Thomas and Mary Fabel's son, also John Fabel, was born seventy miles from Hatfield Peverel in Marham, Norfolk on 7 July 1335, though appears to have grown up mostly in Hatfield Peverel. Thomas Fabel died on 20 May 1349, though his legitimate brother William, his wife Mary and his son John survived the Black Death, and Mary Fabel married a second husband called Ralph Picot or Pycot.[18] At the time of his father's death, John Fabel, who was not yet 14, had gone to live in the household of a knight called Robert Marny or Marenny, who was appointed as his guardian and custodian of John's lands during his minority.

Sir Robert Marny, born in *c.* 1319 and thus about 30 during the pandemic, held the Essex manor of Layer Marney, three miles from the Baynard family's home in Messing and twelve miles from Hatfield Peverel. He was a rather violent, unpleasant character who was frequently imprisoned for assault and robbery, though Edward III, who seems to have had a soft spot for him, repeatedly pardoned him for his felonies.[19] In April 1353, the teenaged John Fabel complained that Robert Marny and his associates 'took him by force' at Witham in Essex and imprisoned him, and subsequently compelled him 'by force and duress' to sign over all his inheritance from his late father to Marny. One of the places where they held him captive was Layer Marney. Lawsuits dragged on well into the 1360s, though the unfortunate John Fabel never managed to regain his inheritance, and died in obscurity at an unknown date. Robert Marny made something of a habit of abducting young heirs and taking over their lands. John Blome died in May 1348, and John Upton, one of his tenants in Kingsey (in Buckinghamshire near the Oxfordshire border), also died that year leaving a 2-year-old son, William. Marny 'abducted the aforesaid heir from the king's wardship and still has him in custody' in 1357.[20] Ultimately Marny got away with this as well and lived to a ripe old age, finally dying in 1400 when he must have been a good 80 years old.

Robert Marny was not the only person who tried to take advantage of the chaos in England in the late 1340s and afterwards, and who profited from bereft and vulnerable orphans (though many others did their best to look after young survivors; see Chapter 20 below). John Parmenter, who came from York, moved – as so many others did in the fourteenth century – to London, where he raised a family. John and his wife, whose name is unknown, died during the plague in 1349, as did all their children except one, their daughter Ellen. Robert Haugham, whom John had appointed as his executor, died too. Robert's own executor, Robert Wodham, appeared before the mayor of London's court on 7 September 1349, charged with the theft of £30 in cash, a signet ring and other items that had belonged to the Parmenters and should have passed to their only surviving child Ellen.

A man named William Spershore, who had probably been a colleague of John Parmenter and his wife Joan had taken the matter to the authorities, and in December 1349 the Spershore couple were appointed as Ellen Parmenter's guardians.[21] Some adults sought to steal goods and property that rightfully belonged to orphaned children, but it is heartening to realise that many others looked out for the children's welfare, and that the authorities, even during or shortly after the greatest pandemic in English history, intervened to protect the children's interests.

Another Essex victim of the Black Death was John Helyon of Helions Bumpstead ('Bomestede Helioun'), who died either on 23 May or 18 June 1349. Born on 14 September 1321, John was 27 at the time of his death, and his wife Agnes was either already dead or also succumbed to the plague. Their son Henry, named after John's father (*c.* 1299–1332), was born on *c.* 24 June 1346 and was not yet 3 years old when he lost his father. On 1 May 1347, rather intriguingly, Edward III had ordered the then 25-year-old John Helioun to appear before the king's council to 'answer certain things which will be laid against him'. John failed to appear, and on 16 July 1347 the king ordered him to be arrested and brought before Chancery to 'answer for his contempt and for other things laid against him'. John's son Henry lived until 1391, and in turn named his son after his father: John Helyon the younger was born on 14 February 1379 in Chrishall, eighteen miles from Helions Bumpstead.[22]

Another plague victim in Essex was Richard Wynchestre of Great Parndon, who died on 8 May 1349. Richard was the son of the interestingly named Taillefer or Taylifer Wynchestre, and was married to Joan, who lived until August 1361. Richard and Joan had three children who were still very young when they lost their father: John, born in *c.* 1345, who outlived his father but died before his mother, Meliora, born in *c.* 1342, and Katherine, born in *c.* 1344, both of whom were still alive in 1361.[23] The Benstede family were lords of the manor of Great Parndon, and John Benstede, who was born on 14 July 1332 and lost his 21-year-old father Edmund in early 1334, lived through the plague, as did his mother Maud. John later had two sons, John and Edward, born close together in 1353 and 1354, and died in 1358. Maud Benstede, widow of Edmund, outlived her son John by more than twenty years, and her grandson Edward Benstede died in October 1432 in his late 70s.[24]

The plague was perhaps past its worst in Essex and Kent by mid-August 1349 as, on Saturday 15 August, a group of more than a dozen men met in Colchester to hold John de Burgh's proof of age: they demonstrated that he was born in Great Oakley, five miles from Harwich, on 5 February 1328.[25] And Henry atte Wode (i.e., Atwood in modern spelling) of Hatfield Regis, three miles from White Roding, also known as Hatfield Broad Oak, who made his will on 8 May 1349 evidently in expectation of imminent death, lived through the pandemic. He died in October 1357, survived by his daughter Elizabeth and perhaps also by his other children Alice, Katherine and William.[26]

The Black Death was, however, to take the life of one of the most remarkable men of the fourteenth century. Thomas Bradwardine was born around 1300, probably in Sussex, and first appears on record as a fellow of Balliol College, Oxford in 1321. He had obtained his Master of Arts degree by 1323, when he moved to Merton College, and was later a Doctor of Theology and professor of divinity. As his entry in the Oxford Dictionary of National Biography states, Thomas Bradwardine 'continued the combination of mathematician, scientist, and theologian characteristic of Oxford since the time of Robert Grosseteste (d. 1253)'. Thomas wrote works on geometry, arithmetic, motion and logical fallacies, and his *Tractatus de proportionibus*, published in 1328 when he was almost certainly not yet 30 years old, is considered particularly significant in the history of mathematical physics. Thomas also composed works of theology such as *De causa Dei* in 1344, and entered royal service: he was an eyewitness to Edward III's victory over the French at the battle of Crécy in 1346, and a few weeks later preached a sermon in English before the king and a group of noblemen after Lord Neville and Lord Percy's victory over a Scottish army at Neville's Cross.[27] John Ufford, who had been archbishop of Canterbury since September 1348 following the death of the aged John Stratford, died on 20 May 1349. He was very briefly succeeded by Thomas Bradwardine, who was appointed on 4 June and died on 26 August from the plague. Simon Islip from Oxfordshire, a fellow of Merton College and a doctor of canon and civil law, was subsequently appointed.

John Segrave of Folkestone in Kent died on 8 July, and his widow, whose name is not recorded, gave birth to his posthumous daughter Mary on 7 August. Mary was still alive when John's inquisition post mortem was held, but died on 25 August 1349 at the age of 18 days, and the little girl's heir was named as her paternal grandmother Juliana Sandwich's cousin Nicholas Sandwich. John Segrave was 29 years old when his father died in October 1343, so was 34 or 35 when he died in July 1349. In February 1351, his heir was named as his cousin John, Lord Segrave (b. 1315), husband of the king's cousin Margaret, countess of Norfolk.[28]

Two sisters, Katherine Gower, born on 25 November 1340, and Joan Gower, born on 22 June 1342, were growing up in Brabourne in Kent. They were both named after their godmothers – Katherine Strathbogie, countess of Atholl, and Joan Passele – and Katherine Gower also happened to be born on the feast day of St Katherine, 25 November. Their village, Brabourne, belonged to the Strathbogies or Strabolgies, a family of Scottish origin who claimed the earldom of Atholl in Scotland and used the title, though, as they lived in England, it was merely an empty claim. David Strathbogie, titular earl of Atholl, born to Scottish parents in Newcastle-upon-Tyne on 1 February 1309, was killed at the battle of Culblean in Aberdeenshire on 30 November 1335. His widow Katherine Strathbogie née Beaumont (b. *c.* mid-1310s), Katherine Gower's godmother, was the sister-in-law of Edward III's kinsman Henry of Grosmont, earl of Lancaster, Leicester, Derby and Lincoln, and the eldest daughter of Alice Beaumont, titular countess of Buchan (d. 9 July 1349). The Gower sisters' father Robert Gower died not long before 6 August 1349, and Katherine Strathbogie was granted custody of the two girls.[29] Katherine Gower died around Christmas 1358, not long after she turned 18. Her sister Joan married William Neve of Weeting in Norfolk, and was still alive in 1367.[30] Brabourne had meadows called *Saltwodemede*, *Parkemede* and *Gavelmede*, and some of its residents who lived through the first pandemic of the plague were John Hamond, who became a baker in Wye five miles from Ashford, Roger Edmund, who became a baker in Hythe on the Kent coast, John Lefsone, Philip Pikehare, Robert Westbech and William Wybarn.[31]

Thomas Deen of Boughton Malherbe in Kent was born on 26 December 1319 as the son of William Deen (d. 1341) and Elizabeth Gatton. Thomas and his wife Martha had four daughters: Benedicta, born *c.* 1344, Margaret, born *c.* 1345, Martha, born *c.* 1347 and Joan, born *c.* 1348. Thomas died not long before 12 May 1349, aged 29; his inquisition post mortem states that he died on 18 May, but the writ to hold the inquisition was issued on

12 May, so he was obviously dead by then. His widow Martha died before 7 June, and, horribly, all four of their daughters, aged 5, 4, 2 and 1, were dead by 30 June 1349.[32] There is no way of knowing if all the little girls died of plague, or if perhaps some of them died of dehydration, starvation or neglect, alone in the house with their parents dead. Even if neighbours were still alive and tried to look after them, if there was no other woman nearby who was breastfeeding an infant, it must have proved impossible to keep Joan, the 1-year-old, alive. During the pandemic, it is likely that older siblings looked after younger siblings in some cases after their parents died, but in the case of the Deen family, the eldest daughter, Benedicta, was still only 5 years old, and was surely far too little to do much to help her younger sisters. An entire family of two parents and four children were wiped out in mere weeks, and the true chilling horror of the Black Death reveals itself in the fate of the young Deen family of Kent.

Chapter 15

Lincolnshire and Cambridgeshire

William Thorney was born in the early 1300s in Whaplode Drove, a small village in southern Lincolnshire nine miles from the village of Thorney over the border in Cambridgeshire, from where William's family presumably took their name. He was the son of Ivo and Christine Thorney, and had a brother Thomas and a sister Lettice, who married Stephen Bageneye and had daughters Alice, Joan and Maud. William had other relatives in Crowland, six miles from Whaplode Drove, and at some point he acquired a plot of land twelve miles away near Wisbech. The plot was called *Brodedrove*, and today there are still places in and around Wisbech called Broad Drove. The Thorney family were poor, but, sometime before 1323, William and his brother Thomas had the great good fortune to be taken on as apprentices by John Grantham, who also came from Lincolnshire and became a successful and wealthy pepperer (a spice merchant) in London. John served as mayor of London from October 1328 to October 1329, and died in 1345.[1] William Thorney became very well-off after he completed his apprenticeship with John Grantham: in his will, he left large bequests of money to his 'poor kinsfolk' in Crowland and his native Whaplode Drove, and by January 1345 was wealthy enough to be able to lend £250 (something like half a million pounds in modern values) to the abbot of Crowland.[2]

By the early 1330s, William was living in the parish of St Mary Aldermary in London with a widow named Joan Armenters. He served as one of the two sheriffs of London in 1339/40, and in the early 1340s was elected alderman of Coleman Street ward.[3] In August 1340, during William's tenure as sheriff, a massive argument took place in the city between groups of fishmongers and skinners, and a fishmonger was stabbed to death by a group of skinners. Violent quarrels between members of the London guilds were not uncommon, but this one blew up into something deeply serious when a fishmonger named Thomas Haunsard threatened the mayor of London, Andrew Aubrey

(d. 1358), with a drawn sword, and Thomas's associate John Brewere hit the mayor's sergeant Simon Berkyng on the head and felled him to the ground so that 'his life is despaired of'. Edward III was away from England at the time and emergency measures were in place in London during the king's absence overseas. Thomas Haunsard and John Brewere admitted their guilt to an assembly of more than 500 men and were sentenced to be beheaded. They were taken to Cheapside forthwith, where William Thorney and his fellow sheriff Roger Forsham carried out the executions next to the stone cross there (demolished in 1643). King Edward indemnified them in June 1341, stating that he had 'charged them to keep the peace in his absence and to inflict swift punishment on any who broke the same'.[4]

At some point, William married a woman called Joan – probably not the same person as Joan Armenters, his landlady or lover in the early 1330s – and their son John was born in 1347. William Thorney made two wills on 20 June 1349 and died before 27 July, when one of the wills was proved. His wife Joan was already dead, and their son John was barely 2 years old when he was orphaned; he was looked after by his uncle Thomas Thorney, and came of age in 1368. John Thorney was still alive in 1401 when he was 54 and married to a woman called Isabel.[5] His father left him numerous household goods and a book in Latin called *The Proverbs of Solomon*, and William left his plot of land near Wisbech to his three nieces, his late sister Lettice Bageneye's daughters Alice Saleman, Joan Rolle and Maud Bageys.

Alice South was born in the Lincolnshire village of Withern, nine miles from Louth, on 6 February 1343, the only child of Robert South and Joan Saltfletby. The family owned a house and land in Strubby, ten acres of meadow in Mabelthorpe on the Lincolnshire coast and a homestead – where Alice was probably born – with ten acres of meadow and 30 acres of arable land in Withern. Robert South died on 3 June 1349 and his wife Joan just fifteen days later on 18 June. Six-year-old Alice was suddenly orphaned. Thankfully her maternal grandfather Robert Saltfletby of Habrough in Lincolnshire, born in 1299, lived through the Black Death and was alive until August 1356, and his son John (b. *c.* 1326), Alice's uncle, survived as well. Robert divided his property equally between his son John and his granddaughter Alice South.

Despite Alice's youth, within three weeks of her father's death she was married to Hugh Cumberworth, who was about 15 years old to her 6 and whose father William Cumberworth died on 25 July 1349 a few weeks after Alice's parents. In fairness, this terribly early marriage was surely intended to protect Alice and her inheritance. The abduction and forced marriage of underage heirs, both female and male, was shockingly common in fourteenth-century England, even though it was potentially punishable by life imprisonment. The village of Cumberworth is nine miles from Alice's home in Withern, and Eudo Doget, another resident of Cumberworth, died on 10 August 1349.[6]

The Saltfletby/South Family of Lincolnshire

Herbert Saltfletby (*c.* 1270–1309) m. Isabel

|

Robert Saltfletby (1299–1356)

|

Joan (d. 1349) m. Robert South (d. 1349)　　John Saltfletby (*c.* 1326–after 1356)

|

Alice South (b. 1343) m. Hugh Cumberworth (b. *c.* 1334)

In the hamlet of Tothby, six miles from Cumberworth, Gilbert Ward died on 28 September 1349. He had two daughters, 6-year-old Margaret and 3-year-old Maud. Maud was still alive in 1363, though her older sister had died by then.[7] In nearby Beesby, Gilbert Ulseby died on 10 August 1349, though his son Hugh, born *c.* April 1334, survived.[8] Forty-five miles southwest of Cumberworth, in Kelby near Ancaster, John Keleby was born on 19 May 1329 as the son of Hugh and Isabel Keleby, and died at the age of 20 on Monday, 3 August 1349. John's sister Alice died in 1353, though their cousins Agnes Keleby, born in April 1334, and her sister Alice, born in July 1337, lived longer.[9]

In Pickworth, a few miles from Grantham, Adam Pikworth died on 7 July 1349 'in the pestilence', his son William Pikworth died on 12 July, and William's cousin Robert Saperton died on 3 August. Robert's son John Saperton, born in *c.* 1346, was heir to his father and his kinsmen Adam and William, and was alive in 1358.[10] Sir John Paynell of Boothby Pagnell, seven miles from Pickworth, was married to Cecily, and their son John the younger was born on 2 May 1345, presumably in the manor-house in Boothby Pagnell that was built around 1200 and still exists. He was baptised in the church of St Andrew in Boothby Pagnell, which also still exists, by the local parson, Richard Pynzon. John Paynell the father died on 25 July 1349 when his son was 4 years old, and seventeen years later, eleven local residents took part in John the son's proof of age. One was Geoffrey Kebet, born in *c.* 1322, who in 1345 had recently moved to the hamlet of Humby near Boothby Pagnell from Bingham near Nottingham, where Laurence Pavely (see Chapter 11) was born in July 1327. Another was William Kyrnell, whose brother Edmund was born on 3 May 1345, the day after John Paynell. John Paynell was raised by his mother Cecily and her second husband Thomas Botheby. In 1376, John witnessed a grant alongside Andrew Luttrell (1313–90), a knight of Lincolnshire whose father Geoffrey (1276–1345) commissioned the Luttrell Psalter.[11]

John Seymour of Hardwick near Wellingborough in Northamptonshire died on Tuesday, 14 July 1349 at the age of about 34. His first son John the younger was born in Hardwick on 6 January 1337, and the boy's godfathers were William Yonge, then aged 23, and John Nichol, aged 29, who were both still alive in the late 1350s. His second son was William Seymour, just under two years younger than his brother, born on *c.* 24 December 1338. John the father appears to have been, if the dates were correctly recorded, 'sick unto death' on Friday 3 July, eleven days before he died. His sister Elizabeth and both of his sons lived into adulthood, though John Seymour the younger died in 1362 when he was 25.[12]

In Hogsthorpe, seven miles north of Skegness, Robert Cracroft died on 10 August 1349. His son John was born in the village on 13 March 1335, so was 14 when he lost his father. John Cracroft was named after his godfather John Beseby, whose son Peter, born *c.* 1310, was still alive in 1358. A few weeks after his son was born in 1335, Robert Cracroft went on pilgrimage to the shrine of St Thomas Becket in Canterbury with two friends, Philip Thoresthorp and Eudo Billesby, 'in fulfilment of a vow on account of danger in coming from assizes at Lincoln in thunder and lightning, from which they were in fear of death'. Three of the jurors who took part in John's proof of age in 1358 remembered his birth because at the beginning of August 1335, a few months after he was born, 'there was a great inundation of sea water' that broke the sea walls at Mablethorpe and drowned livestock. Another juror was Robert Alisonson, born in *c.* 1306. His last name means that he was the son of a woman named Alison – itself a diminutive of the name Alis or Alice – and that he was illegitimate.[13]

Chapter 16

Huntingdonshire, Rutland, East Anglia

Eleanor Stokes of Boughton in Huntingdonshire, a deserted medieval village that lay between Huntingdon and St Neots and no longer exists, died on 13 July 1349. Eleanor left a son, Thomas Wauton, who was about 30 in 1349 and married to a woman called Amice, and she also had three daughters from her second marriage to Nicholas Gamage: Margaret or Margery, Elizabeth and Joan. Eleanor's brother-in-law John Fyn, widower of her sister Margaret Stokes, had died a few weeks earlier on 5 June, also in Boughton, and her second husband Nicholas Gamage is almost certainly the man of this name who died in late January or early February 1349 and is mentioned in Chapter 4 above. Although Eleanor was married twice, to men called Wauton and Gamage, she used the surname of her father, John Stokes.[1] Robert Vernon of Abbots Ripton in Huntingdonshire died on 17 June 1349; his son Robert was born in the village on 1 March 1346, and was still alive decades later.[2] John Deene of Upwood a few miles from Huntingdon died on 11 September 1349. His son John the younger was barely 9 years old at the time, and himself died in the early summer of 1354, outlived by his aunt Ada Deene and his cousin John Neville, son of his father's other sister Margaret Deene.[3]

Mary Curzon, whose family came from the village of Ingham a few miles northeast of Norwich, died on 24 July 1349. Born in 1335 or 1336, Mary was only in her early teens when she died, though, despite her youth, she was no stranger to loss. She had already lost both her parents, John Curzon and Elizabeth Ingham, and was a widow; her husband Stephen Tumby died sometime before she did, perhaps also in the pestilence. Mary's maternal grandfather Sir Oliver Ingham (*c.* 1287–1344) enjoyed a long career in royal service, though was temporarily imprisoned by Edward III in October 1330 when the young king overthrew his mother Isabella of France and her ally Roger Mortimer, earl of March – father of Blanche, Lady Grandison and Agnes, countess of Pembroke – who had ruled the kingdom during his minority. Another victim of the plague was Mary Curzon's uncle-in-law Roger Lestrange, husband of her mother's sister Joan Ingham, who died on 2 August 1349. Mary's grandmother Elizabeth Zouche, Oliver Ingham's widow, outlived her and died on 11 October 1350.[4]

The Ingham Family of Norwich

Oliver Ingham (*c.* 1287–1344) m. Elizabeth Zouche (d. 1350)
| |
Elizabeth Ingham m. John Curzon   Joan Ingham m. 1) Roger Lestrange (1301–49)
| m. 2) Miles Stapleton (*c.* 1320–64)
Mary Curzon (1335/36–49)
m. Stephen Tumby (d. 1349 or before)

William Grymbaud of Diddington in Huntingdonshire died on 9 May 1349. He was 2 years old in March 1327 when he lost his father, so was 24 when he died, and his son Robert was 5.[5] Aubrey Wittlebury of Whissendine in Rutland, between Melton Mowbray and Oakham, died on 13 June 1349, though his mother Katherine and his wife Joan, and his and Joan's three sons, survived. Their eldest son Thomas, 22 years old in 1349, died in 1353; their second son William became a monk at Peterborough Abbey in June 1353 at almost the same time that his brother Thomas died; and their third son John was born in Whissendine on 20 July 1333. Aubrey's father John Wittlebury had been murdered in July 1336, shortly before his grandson John's third birthday. When John Wittlebury the grandson proved his age in August 1354, Whissendine resident Thomas Thop declared that the infant spent the first year of his life in the home of his parents Joan and Aubrey then 'for two years following at the house of Roger Balle in the same [Whissendine] to be nursed'. William Chaumberleyn remembered young John's birth because the month before, in June 1333, he took part in an archery competition and was given a barbed arrow as the best archer.[6]

Margaret Swynford of Great Stukeley in Huntingdonshire died on Monday, 27 July 1349. She was married to Thomas FitzEustace and they had a daughter Joan, who was not named as the heir to Margaret's 'ruinous' house in the village, presumably because she was already dead. Margaret's nephew William Swynford and his wife Eleanor already had daughters Isabel and Elizabeth, and Eleanor was pregnant during the pandemic; she gave birth to their son Thomas Swynford on 31 October 1349. As male heirs took precedence over their older sisters by the law of primogeniture, and as

Margaret's daughter Joan FitzEustace must have been dead, little Thomas became heir to his great-aunt Margaret's house in Great Stukeley. As well as living through the horrors of the plague while pregnant, the unfortunate Eleanor Swynford had to contend with the death of her husband. William Swynford died near Smithfield, London on 24 June 1349, perhaps of the plague, which was then raging through the city. His son was born four months later.[7]

Edward III's cousin Alice of Norfolk was probably born in 1324, and was the younger sister of Margaret, countess of Norfolk, who died in 1399 at the age of 76 or 77. They were the daughters and heirs of Edward I's son Thomas of Brotherton, earl of Norfolk (1300–38), believed to have been the child cured of smallpox by John Gaddesden in the early 1300s. Alice gave birth to her fifth and youngest child, Joan Montacute, in Bungay, Suffolk on 2 February 1349.[8] Alice's husband Edward Montacute was the brother of the late earl of Salisbury, William Montacute (d. 1344), and uncle of the earl of Salisbury who proved his age in 1349. None of the jurors at Joan Montacute's proof of age (held in Bungay on 7 February 1363) mentioned the pestilence when stating the reasons why they remembered the date of Joan's birth, though Hugh Graunt said that his son Nicholas broke his thigh in late June 1349, and Thomas Crane, who was about 24 in 1349, set off on pilgrimage to Santiago de Compostela at the beginning of August that year. It seems incredible that he was willing to travel overseas at such a time.

Alice of Norfolk and her daughter Joan Montacute were not destined to enjoy long and happy lives and, horrifically, Alice was beaten to death by her husband and two of his retainers. It appears that the attack took place in June 1351, and that Alice lingered for a few months, perhaps in a coma, before finally succumbing to her injuries in late 1351 or early 1352.[9] Edward III did not punish Edward Montacute, though he did send Alice's two youngest daughters to live with their long-lived grandmother Elizabeth Montacute née Montfort rather than leaving them with their father. Of Alice's five children, the three eldest died in their teens or younger, and her second youngest child, Maud Montacute, became abbess of Barking Abbey in Essex (a position reserved for women of noble birth). In or before 1362, Joan Montacute married the much older William Ufford, earl of Suffolk. On 14 February 1363, even though she had only turned 14 years old twelve days before, Joan was said to be pregnant by her husband, who was almost 25.[10]

She died sometime before 1382, with no surviving children. Her wife-killing father Edward Montacute and his baby son from his second marriage died less than three months apart in 1361.[11] It is possible, though not certain, that they were both victims of the second pandemic of the Black Death.

Isabel Stanton of East Carleton, six miles southwest of Norwich, died on 16 August 1349. Born in *c.* 1311, she was about 37 or 38 when she died, and was the only child of William Florence (d. 1333) and the widow of Geoffrey Stanton. Isabel and Geoffrey's son Thomas Stanton was born in Stanton, Suffolk on 16 June 1337, and was still alive in early 1368.[12] Two days after Isabel's death, 25 miles away in Stanford, Norfolk, John Clere proved with the aid of a dozen jurors that he was now 21 years old and had been born in the nearby village of Sturston on 14 July 1328. Both of these places, Stanford and Sturston, are now uninhabited after being taken over by the British army as a training area during the Second World War, and are still used as such. John Clere inherited the manor of Sturston (then called Striston or Strystone) from his father Edmund, who was murdered by one Geoffrey Beman when John was only a week old. The unfortunate John also lost his mother, Isabel, not long before 28 May 1331, and was an orphan before he was 3 years old.[13] John Honeworth of Bodham near Cromer died on 7 September 1349, though his widow Margaret or Margery was still alive in the 1360s. Their three children, William (born *c.* 1338), Margaret (born *c.* 1340) and Katherine (born *c.* 1342), survived too. John Honeworth was born in Bodham on 25 March 1309, so was 40 when he died.[14]

In the Middle Ages, Dunwich on the Suffolk coast was a large and thriving port, though it is now merely a tiny village. Terrible storms in 1286/87 destroyed much of the harbour, and the port's decline was accelerated by the first pandemic of the Black Death. In 1354, an inquisition found that Dunwich was 'impoverished and destroyed' and that much of the town was now under water, with the rest in a ruinous state. There had once been over 2,000 men 'at scot and lot' in the town, but since 1349 this number had dwindled to a mere 47 men, who had been 'impoverished by the plague'.[15]

A Norfolk couple, John and Elizabeth Bardolf, had a son in 1349: William Bardolf was born in Wormegay near King's Lynn (then called 'Lenne') on 21 October.[16] William's mother Elizabeth Bardolf née Damory was the younger half-sister of Isabella Verdon, Lady Ferrers, who died on 25 July 1349 while Elizabeth was pregnant. William's father John Bardolf employed a chamberlain, Richard Rysyng, who was in such a hurry to ride to William's godfather to inform him of the boy's birth that he fell from his horse and broke his right leg – though he survived the traumatic accident and was still alive decades later. William Bardolf lost both parents by the time he was 14 and died in 1386; his son Thomas Bardolf, born in December 1369, died in 1408 while taking part in the Percy Rebellion against Edward III's grandson Henry IV.

Chapter 17

Yorkshire (1)

The plague reached Yorkshire by the third week of July 1349. Considering how sparsely populated the north of England was in the fourteenth century – York, with somewhere around 15,000 inhabitants, was by far its biggest settlement – the county of Yorkshire suffered terribly. Roger Basy of Bilbrough, southwest of York, was an early victim in the county: he died on 19 July 1349, leaving his 11-year-old brother Richard and their illegitimate half-brother William Basy, who joined the Church and was alive in 1366.[1] John Cave of Middleton on the Wolds in the East Riding was another early victim, dying on 23 July 1349. His wife Isabel was already dead, and their son John the younger, born in Middleton on 20 December 1332, survived. Other Middleton residents who lived through the plague and were alive in the mid-1350s were John Lyndale, William Ward and Richard of London, who had evidently moved from London to the rural north of England (or perhaps his parents had). John Cave, born in 1332 and a survivor of the Black Death, had a son, or perhaps grandson, born in *c.* 1379 and also called John Cave, whose son, Robert, was born in 1414. This younger John Cave was still alive in 1435, aged about 56.[2]

Richard Rolle, the mystic who left Oxford after a religious conversion and returned to his native Yorkshire to preach, died on 30 September 1349 at Hampole Priory northwest of Doncaster.[3] Another well-known Yorkshireman who died during the plague was Thomas, Lord Wake, a landowner in Yorkshire, Lincolnshire and Cumberland. He died in Chesterfield, Derbyshire on 30 May at the age of 51, and was buried at Haltemprice Priory close to Hull, which he himself had founded a few years earlier. The prior of Haltemprice was also a casualty of the plague, several months later. As Thomas Wake had no children from his marriage of thirty-three years to Blanche of Lancaster, eldest of Henry of Grosmont's six sisters, his heir was his older sister Margaret, dowager countess of Kent. She was the mother of the king's cousin John, earl of Kent, who had married Elisabeth von Jülich the year before. Countess Margaret survived her brother by four months and died on 29 September 1349, the day before Richard Rolle.[4] The marriage of Margaret's daughter Joan of Kent to William Montacute, earl of Salisbury, was annulled in 1349 and, though Margaret could not have known it, Joan would marry her final husband the prince of Wales a few years later and Margaret would be the grandmother of a king of England, Richard II (born 1367). Margaret's sister-in-law Blanche of Lancaster, born at the start of the 1300s, did not die until 1380, having outlived all six of her younger siblings.

The Paynells were a family originally from the Dorset/Wiltshire area who also held lands in Yorkshire and Lincolnshire. Philip Paynell was born in Wiltshire in August 1269 and was named after his great-uncle and godfather Philip Basset, after whose family the Wiltshire villages of Wootton Bassett, Berwick Bassett and Winterbourne Bassett are named. Philip Paynell was the heir of his childless older brother John when the latter died aged 24 in 1287 (John Paynell's widow Amabilla died at what must have been an advanced age in 1349). Philip's wife Elizabeth gave birth to their son, John Paynell, on Christmas Eve in 1296, and John, though born in Dorset, spent most of his life in the north of England and married a woman called Juliana. Their first daughter, Elizabeth Paynell, was probably born in March 1317, and their second, Margery, was born in Drax, a few miles from Selby between Leeds and Hull, in September 1319.

The Paynell Family of Wiltshire and Yorkshire

John Paynell (d. 1275) m. Katherine Periton (d. 1296)

Philip (1269–99) m. Elizabeth (d. 1344) — John (1263–87) m. Amabilla (d. 1349)

John Paynell (1296–1325) m. Juliana (d. 1333)

Margery (1319–49) m. John Pouger (d. 1349) — Elizabeth (1317–72) m. 1) Richard Gascrik (d. 1347); m. 2) John Barton (d. 1348/49); m. 3) Thomas Fulnetby (d. 1372)

John Pouger (1336–1405) — John Gascrik (b. *c.* 1335, d. after 1347)

John Pouger (*c.* 1381–1414)

Henry Pouger (*c.* 1410–20) m. Isabel — Joan Pouger m. John Sotille

The two Paynell sisters lost their father very young when John passed away in March 1325 at the age of 28, and their mother Juliana died in 1333 when they were still in their teens. They did, however, have their paternal grandmother Elizabeth Paynell, who outlived her husband Philip by forty-five years and died in November 1344, and their great-aunt Amabilla, who died on 4 July 1349 during the Black Death when she must have been at least in her mid-70s and was perhaps over 80. Elizabeth Paynell the granddaughter married Richard Gascrik, and her younger sister Margery was married to John Pouger or Poucher of West Rasen, Lincolnshire by December 1334. Elizabeth had a son John Gascrik in about 1335, though he must have died young sometime after 1347, and Margery had a son, named John Pouger like his father, who was born in or not long before April 1336. The Gascrik and Pouger cousins surely knew their great-grandmother Elizabeth Paynell, who died in 1344 when they were about 9 and 8, and their great-great-aunt Amabilla.

After losing her first husband Richard Gascrik on 18 September 1347 when she was 30 years old, the younger Elizabeth Paynell married her second husband John Barton with what seems, by the standards of the time, to be indecent haste: they were already wed by 4 November 1347. This second marriage cannot have lasted long, and by 28 August 1349 Elizabeth was married to her third husband Thomas Fulnetby, who, like Elizabeth's brother-in-law John Pouger, came from West Rasen in Lincolnshire. Elizabeth and Margery inherited 'an old hall on the north side of the church' in West Rasen, as well as three cottages there, some pastureland and ponds.

Margery Pouger née Paynell died on 10 July 1349, two months before her thirtieth birthday and six days after her great-aunt Amabilla finally passed away. Margery's widower John outlived her by a month and died on 12 August 1349. Their son John Pouger the younger was 13 when he lost both his parents, though his aunt Elizabeth Paynell and her third husband Thomas Fulnetby both lived until 1372. It may be that Elizabeth's second husband John Barton also died in the pestilence, and perhaps that her son John Gascrik, who was about 12 when his father died in September 1347, did too; certainly, the boy did not live to be an adult. Elizabeth's nephew John Pouger the younger lived until 1405, when he was close to 70.[5]

At Easter 1369, three men recalled how, just before Christmas in 1348, they had visited the market in Barton-upon-Humber in northern Lincolnshire together. There they met John Cokheved, whose nephew and godson, also John Cokheved, had just been born, and he invited them to his home for a celebratory drink. The infant John's father Hugh Cokheved, a merchant of Barton, held a feast at his own home a few weeks later to celebrate his wife Margaret's purification after childbirth, and paid the minstrels who entertained the guests 40 shillings. Hugh died in July 1351, and his son came of age at the end of the 1360s. John's mother Margaret married a second husband, Robert Gasson, in or before 1357.[6] At the end of 1348 and for a few more months, life continued as normal in Lincolnshire and Yorkshire, but the plague was on its deadly way.

John Merflet of Barton-upon-Humber died on 3 August 1349, and had one child, Hugh Merflet, whose age is not recorded but who was certainly born later than 1340. Hessle – just three miles from Haltemprice Priory, where Lord Wake was buried – is now a suburb of Hull and close to the Humber Bridge, on the other side of the River Humber from Barton. Alan Moigne died in Hessle two days before John Merflet, on 1 August 1349, leaving a 13-year-old son named William.[7] John Constable and his wife Aubrey or Albreda lived in Halsham, a village in the area of Yorkshire called Holderness, close to the North Sea and a few miles east of Hull; they also owned meadow and pasture 'for four fat cows' in nearby Ottringham. John was the son of Robert Constable and Avice Lasceles and was born around 1303/04; he was said to be 32 when his father died in early 1336. His and Aubrey's son John the younger was born in Halsham on 13 October 1336, nine months after his grandfather Robert Constable's death. In the late 1350s, one Robert Lorimer recalled that, while riding through Halsham in October 1336, he had seen 'many men, women and children … rejoicing and praising God' when young John was born.

John Constable the father's inquisition post mortem says that he died around sunset on 17 September 1349, and was 'afflicted with great weakness for four days preceding, at the time of the mortality then raging in those parts'. Several hours before he died, 'about that hour of the day called *Midovernone*' (mid-afternoon), John, though 'languishing in extremis', was sufficiently *compos mentis* to set his seal to a charter relating to the custody of his possessions. Aubrey Constable had married her second husband, John Sturmy, by 11 March 1350, and her son, aged 12 and 11 months when he lost his father to the Black Death, was still alive in 1402, well into his 60s.[8]

Holderness and the area around Hull suffered terribly during the Black Death. Benedict Gummer states that 'almost thirty years' worth of wills were proved in this terrible year of 1349' in that part of England.[9] John Hunteplace of South Frodingham, near Patringham in Holderness, was one of the earliest victims in the area, passing away on 24 July; Robert Upsale, a merchant of Hull, died on 1 August; Ingelram Ingram of Preston in Holderness, who was around 40 years old, died on 4 August 1349, though his son Robert, who was about 22, survived; Isabel, daughter of John of Preston in Holderness, died on 6 August; Stephen Haukyn also of Preston died on 12 August; John Wyveton of Wyton, three miles north of Preston, died on 31 August; and Roger Gylt of Sproatley, a mile from Wyton, died on 31 July. Geoffrey Redmar of Out Newton on the coast of Holderness died on 29 August, and Alice atte See and her son John atte See of nearby Redmar – a settlement which no longer exists – died on 6 August and 15 September respectively. Adam Dyk of Coniston (a village near Hull, not the place of the same name in the Lake District) died on 4 August; John Walcotes of Thorngumbald died on 25 August; Nicholas Thorne of East Newton on the Holderness coast died on 26 August; Beatrice Burton of Burton Pidsea died on 30 August; John Thornton of Rysome died on 6 September; Alice Crokhowe of Tunstall on the coast died on 13 August; and John Pensthorp of Pensthorpe died on 19 or 22 August, and his father Ralph died too. The village of Pensthorpe is now, like Redmar, a lost settlement. Mabel St Martin of Hollym in Holderness died on 5 September, though her adult daughters Isabel and Alice survived, and John Wake also of Hollym died on 6 August. Another lost settlement of the area was Paulflete or Paghelflete, and William Stellare, who owned a home there, died on 26 July, an early victim of the Black Death in Yorkshire; and another Holderness village that is now lost was Hornsea Burton, where Walter Mapelton died on 1 August.[10] Yet another Holderness village that no longer exists was Alde Ravenser or Old Ravenser, and Stephen Thorp died there on 10 August 1349. He was around 36 when he died, and left a son also called Stephen, who was said to be 13 years old in 1363. Either that date is erroneous, or the younger Stephen was born in 1350 a few months after his father's death.[11]

A manor within the parish of Burstwick, also in Holderness, was called *Bondebrustwyk* or Bond Burstwick in the fourteenth century. Its inhabitants who died in the Black Death included Agnes Helpeston, who died on 24 July

1349, another very early victim; John Goushill on 28 July; William Park on 15 August; William Aumener and Peter Moys both on 20 August; and John Aumener, who died on 6 March 1350, a date when the pestilence was well past its terrible peak but still lingered in parts of the country. John Goushill's son Robert was 6 years old in 1349, William Park's son John was 5, John Aumener's daughter Agnes was 14 and Nicholas Thorne, another victim, had a son John who was just 2 and left three young daughters, Maud, Avice and Elizabeth, as well. Peter Moys had two daughters, Alice and Emma, who were both already dead in 1349 but left children. Peter's granddaughter Beatrice Dyk (b. 1334) later married Robert Aumener, evidently a relative of William Aumener and John Aumener. Unlike them, Robert lived through the plague.[12]

Yet another 1349 death in Holderness was that of Margery Botheby of Camerton, who died on 13 September. Margery's husband Robert had died in December 1324, and their son Thomas (born *c.* 1309) and his wife Eustachia died before Margery. Margery's grandson John Botheby, born in Ryehill near Camerton on 2 February 1338, survived the plague. Nicholas Botheby, a relative of Margery's, perhaps her late husband's brother or her younger son, died on 14 November 1349, and his heir was Margery's grandson John.[13] A few years earlier, Margery Botheby had feuded with Peter Moys, John Goushill, William Aumener and William Park over a sewer that flooded Margery's lands, and which she had blocked up. Now they were all dead in the Black Death.[14]

The death toll in Holderness between July and September 1349 was horrifying, though, thankfully, some residents survived and were still alive in the late 1350s and 1360s, such as Peter Moys' granddaughter Beatrice Aumener née Dyk; Margery Botheby's grandson John Botheby; Joan Thorp of Brandesburton, born in 1340; Edmund Wasteneys, born *c.* 1300; Gerard Grimston of Aldbrough, born *c.* 1308; Hugh Gylt, born *c.* 1311, who lost his father Roger to the pestilence; Thomas Lelle, born in Barmston in 1319, and his son William Lelle, born in 1338; Robert Edenhale, born *c.* 1317, and his wife Alice Charleton; Amand Flinton, born *c.* 1314; and John Sprotle or Sprotteleye (i.e., he came from the village of Sproatley), born *c.* 1300/04. John Sprotle recalled in 1358 how in 1336 he had made a pilgrimage to the shrine of St Thomas Becket in Canterbury, 250 miles away, after recovering from an illness. He lived through the pestilence a few years later, as did his daughter Alice Sprotle, born in June 1340. North of Holderness lies the village of Dringhoe, and Edmund Cauce died there on 8 December 1347. His heir was his son Robert, aged 8 weeks when Edmund's inquisition post mortem was taken on 19 January 1348. Robert was alive on 12 July 1349 but died before 3 September 1349, not yet 2 years old, on which date his older sister Isabel died as well. Edmund Cauce was said to be 25 years old in 1342, so was 30 when he died in late 1347, before the Black Death reached England. His brother John Cauce was about 26 in 1349, and appears to have survived the plague.[15]

Chapter 18

Yorkshire (2)

Thomas Archer, son of John and Joan Archer, was born in Bolton, a village northwest of Pocklington in Yorkshire, on 19 August 1345, and was baptised in nearby Yapham on the day of his birth. His father John Archer died in the pestilence on 25 July 1349, aged about 24, and John's widow Joan was still alive in 1366. Thomas Archer survived as well, as did another child, John atte Essh, born in Bolton around the same time. At Thomas Archer's proof of age held in Pocklington in the autumn of 1366, Richard Veile, then aged about 56, stated that in August 1345 'he had three sons born of his wife', though did not give his wife's name, nor clarify whether any of the triplets survived their birth.[1]

Ralph Arblaster of Great Givendale near Pocklington died on 25 July 1349. Probably born in August 1323, Ralph was 25, almost 26, when he died, and had no children from his marriage to Isabel. His sisters Alice and Agnes were said to be 26 and 24 in 1349; if these ages are correct, Alice must have been Ralph's twin. They were the children of Walter, who died in 1328, and Mariote, who died in 1346 after marrying a second husband named William Bacheler. Alice Arblaster died apparently unmarried in May 1361, and an inquisition states that the few acres of land she had inherited from her brother had lain 'waste and untilled' since his death, an indication of the dearth of people available to work the land since the pestilence. Alice's younger sister Agnes outlived her, and their sister-in-law, Ralph's widow Isabel, was still alive in 1392, having married a second husband, Nicholas Hastings.[2] The name Arblaster originally meant a soldier who used an arbalest, i.e., a crossbow.

Several other Great Givendale residents who lived through the plague as small children and were still alive decades later were Elizabeth Wynestowe, John Holme, Philip Coke, Joan Kelk, William Mareschall, Joan Croke and Ralph Hobkyn, who was born in the village on 13 November 1346 and baptised by Nicholas Wilton, parson of the village church. Ralph's father

William Hobkyn died around the time he was born.[3] Walter Quixley of Great Givendale died on 3 August 1349, a few days after Ralph Arblaster, in his mid or late 40s. In 1364, the two houses Walter had owned were said to be in ruins, presumably because no-one had lived there since the pestilence. He had no children, but his brother John left daughters Maud, born in *c.* 1344 and still alive in 1372, and Agnes, born in *c.* 1346, who died before 1372.[4] Adam Freman was another local victim: he lived in Warter, four and a half miles from Pocklington, and died on 12 August 1349, 'in the pestilence'. His son John, born in 1337, was alive in 1361. An older John Freman also of Warter, presumably a relative of Adam, died on 18 August.[5]

The village of Wharram Percy, twelve miles from Great Givendale, is a DMV or 'deserted medieval village' that is very well-known today. Walter Heslarton owned the manor of Wharram Percy via his wife Eustachia Percy, who inherited it from her parents Peter and Isabel, and died on either 24 August or 9 September 1349. Eustachia was born in *c.* 1312/13, so was in her mid-30s when her husband died. She had a sister Joan, about two years younger than she, who died as a child in *c.* 1324 and was buried in Grimsby, which left Eustachia as sole heir to their father Peter Percy and grandfather Robert Percy. Eustachia gave birth to her son Walter Heslarton the younger around 15 August 1333.[6] On 16 August 1349, just a few days before he died, Eustachia's husband Walter was one of a group of people – including one woman – accused of raiding a house in Normanby near Glentham in Lincolnshire, which belonged to Margaret Beek, and stealing her goods. Eustachia stated in December 1350 that in her widowhood, she was 'broken by age and very feeble' – she was still under 40 years old – and the king appointed three men to be 'guardians and defenders of her and her lands'.[7] Eustachia Heslarton née Percy died in or not long before January 1365, and an inquisition in 1367 found that she 'was an idiot from birth'. In the rather unkind language of the time, this implied some degree of mental incapacity and an inability to take care of oneself or one's property, though Eustachia seems to have managed her affairs perfectly well until she lost her husband in the Black Death, and her son Walter did not take over her lands until after she died, by which time he was over 30.[8]

Robert Frithby of Eddlethorpe in North Yorkshire, seven and a half miles from Wharram Percy, died on 20 August 1349, and his mother Agnes née Houby, widow of John Frithby, died either on 23 September, 27 September or 14 October 1349. Robert's elder son John Frithby, Agnes's grandson, was born in Eddlethorpe on 24 June 1335, and his younger son Edmund was born in *c.* 1339. Fourteen-year-old John was already married in 1349, but he left no children when he died in October 1362; his younger brother Edmund fathered three children before his death in 1375.[9]

A surprisingly large number of babies were born in Upleathem, twelve miles from Middlesbrough, in July 1345 who lived through the plague and were all alive in 1366: Alice Lakenby, Joan Rosele, John Eden, Robert Boynton, Agnes Foulthorp, Thomas Wyles, Thomas Kloket, Agnes Capon and Joan Dalhouse. Another was Thomas Fauconberg, born on 20 July 1345. In 1378, Thomas was imprisoned for treason, accused of joining the French against his native England, and was not released until 1391; his younger brother Roger Fauconberg – another child who lived through the Black Death – complained in 1390 that he had been imprisoned for so long 'that his person is well-nigh brought to nought'. Perhaps as a result of this long incarceration, Thomas was believed to be suffering from mental incapacity: in 1403, it was said that 'he is not of sound mind but enjoys lucid intervals'. Thomas's children from his first marriage predeceased him, and his daughter and heir Joan, from his second marriage, was born in Skelton on 18 October 1406 when he was 61. He died less than a year later on 9 September 1407.[10]

The village of Acklam is in Ryedale, about twelve miles northeast of York, and the pestilence arrived there by 14 August 1349, when Robert Cornwalays died. Robert's son, also Robert, was already dead, and left three children: Isabel, whose date of birth is not recorded, Thomas, who was said to be 2 years old in 1349, and Alice, the eldest sibling, who was born in Acklam on 15 August 1337; her grandfather died in the pestilence the day before she turned 12. Isabel and Thomas Cornwalays died young, perhaps later in 1349, and Alice was still alive in May 1362, not yet married.[11] Other residents of Acklam who survived the pestilence were Juliana Brett, born in August 1337, her older brother John Brett, 13-year-old Robert Crook, born in the village on 9 February 1336, and his parents William Crook and Denise, née Thoraldby. William Crook died in March 1353, and by March 1355 Denise was married to her second husband, John Warthorp. John Warde, who was 12 or 13, was an Acklam resident who died in the pestilence, though his brother Philip, who was about 15, survived. John Ulbright of Acklam married his wife Alice around Easter 1336 when they were both in their teens, and they both survived the plague. Alice died in 1361; John outlived her.[12]

Robert Bustard, who lived in Bishopthorpe, just south of York, died on 19 August 1349, and his mother Maud outlived him by many years and died in early 1366. Robert appears to have been born around 1314 or a little earlier, so was in his mid-30s when he died, and if he ever married, there is no record of it. His only sibling, Joan, had married John Friston, and though she was already dead in 1349, she left three children: Maud, born in 1341 or 1342, who later married John Deyvill of Bilton; Richard Bustard aka Richard Friston – he appears on record with both his father's and his mother's surnames – born in *c.* 1343; and Margaret, born in *c.* 1344, who later married John Clifton. All three children lived through the pandemic, though Richard died in November 1363, aged 20. Maud Deyvill née Friston died on 8 June 1416, aged 74 or 75, and her sister Margaret Clifton née Friston died on 1 June 1422, aged about 78. Except for Robert Bustard's sister Joan Friston née Bustard, who died comparatively young, perhaps in childbirth, the women of his family had long lives. His grandmother Margaret outlived his grandfather by forty-one years and lived long enough to see her great-grandchildren, his mother Maud outlived his father by forty-four years, and his nieces Maud and Margaret lived well into their 70s and survived their brother Richard by fifty-three and fifty-nine years.[13]

Warin Scargill of Ossett between Dewsbury and Wakefield died on 13 September 1349, outlived by his father William (d. *c.* 1352) and his 9-year-old son William the younger, alive in 1380.[14] Robert Langethwayt of Rillington, near Malton, who had a baby daughter named Margaret, died on 20 August 1349, and Ralph Cloughton of Scalby, eighteen miles from Rillington, died on 22 September. His son, also Ralph, was said to be 8 years old in May 1358, so appears to have been born posthumously.[15]

The Bustard Family of Bishopthorpe, Yorkshire

Robert Bustard (*c.* 1250–1302) m. Margaret (d. 1343)

John Bustard (*c.* 1283–1322) m. Maud (d. 1366)

Robert Bustard (*c.* 1314–49) | Joan Bustard (d. before 1349) m. John Friston

Maud (1341/42–1416) m. John Deyvill
Richard Bustard aka Friston (*c.* 1343–63)
Margaret (*c.* 1344–1422) m. John Clifton

Henry FitzHenry was born in Ingleton in the area of the country now called the Yorkshire Dales in the spring of 1344: he was said to be a year and a half old when his father John's inquisition post mortem was held in October 1345. John FitzHenry died on the island of Rhodes on 6 July 1345 on his way to the Holy Land, and news of his death did not reach England until 10 September. Young Henry died on 12 October 1349, aged only 5. His aunt Beatrice, John's sister, and her husband Thomas Fencotes survived the plague, as did Henry's grandmother Joan.[16]

Chapter 19

Westmorland, Cumberland, Northumberland

The plague reached the lightly populated northernmost counties of England – Westmorland and Cumberland in the west and Northumberland in the east – at the start of October 1349. Joan Parvyng of Blackwell near Carlisle in Cumberland, widow of John Pacok and sister of the late Robert Parvyng, died on 1 October 1349. Joan Parvyng and John Pacok had a son called Adam, who was of full age, i.e., at least 21, in 1349, and was, in another example of the often-fluid naming conventions of the era, known both as Adam Pacok and Adam Parvyng. His son Robert, who died in 1405, was known by the name Parvyng. Adam's maternal uncle Robert Parvyng (d. 1343) had no children, and Adam's mother Joan and her sister Emma Scaleby were their brother's heirs. The rest of the Parvyng/Pacok family appear to have survived the pestilence.[1] Robert Raghton of Raughton in Cumberland, eight miles south of Carlisle, died on 3 October 1349. His son Thomas was just 3 years old, born in Carlisle on 14 August 1346, and was alive in the early 1400s.[2]

Robert Botiller of the tiny settlement of King's Meaburn in Westmorland, which even in the twenty-first century has a population of a mere 150 or so, died on 15 October 1349. Robert had seven adult daughters: Joan Heton, Margery Brantingham, Beatrice Laybourne, Ellen Bagley, Maud Hanlaghby, Agnes Prodhomme and Alice Kirkebythore, of whom Agnes and Alice died before their father, leaving children. The other five women survived their father, and John Kirkebythore, son of Robert's daughter Alice and her husband Thomas, proved his age in February 1363: he was born in Kirkby Thore on 6 October 1340, and lost his grandfather a few days after his ninth birthday. John was still alive in February 1392.[3]

John Cudberd of Brougham in Westmorland died on 3 October 1349. He had no children, and his heirs were his nieces Christine, Alice and Joan, the daughters of his late sister Eda, and his 8-year-old great-nephew Adam, grandson of his other late sister Isabel.[4] In the small village of Newbiggin, five miles from Brougham, Robert Crakanthorp died on 4 October, the day after John Cudberd. Robert's wife Emma, heir of the Newbiggin family, died sometime before January 1351 and perhaps also fell victim to the plague. Their son William Crakanthorp was born in 1330 or earlier and, in August 1354, took part in the proof of age of Roger, Lord Clifford, who was born in Westmorland on 20 July 1333. William remembered the date when Roger Clifford was born because two days later the village of Crackenthorpe 'was burned and destroyed by the Scots' (as noted in Chapter 11 above, Edward III defeated a Scottish force at the battle of Halidon Hill near Berwick-on-Tweed on 19 July 1333). William Crakanthorp was still alive in February 1368, when he was replaced as coroner of Westmorland on the grounds of being 'insufficiently qualified'. His Crakanthorp descendants still lived in the area in the fifteenth century.[5]

Thomas Dolfanby of Bramwra near Penrith died on 10 October 1349, though his brother William and William's son John survived.[6] In Strickland Ketel near Kendal, about twenty-eight miles south of Penrith, William Alaynson died on 20 October 1349. William was a widower, and his elder daughter Christina was already dead, but she left a 3-year-old daughter Sybil, and Sybil's aunt Elizabeth Alaynson, William's younger daughter, was alive in 1357 though was still only 18 years old then.[7] John Hotounrof was born in Hutton Roof near Kirkby Lonsdale on 20 March 1345, and lived through the pestilence as a 4-year-old. People who lived in and around the Westmorland town of Penrith who also survived the pandemic of 1349 and were still alive in the late 1360s were Alice Lenton, Isabel Stapleton and Isabel Beauchamp, all born in the mid-1340s, and their fathers John Lenton, William Stapleton and Roger Beauchamp, all born in the early to mid-1320s, the brothers William and Thomas Hoton, Roger Salkeld, who was born around 1317, and Gilbert Suthayk, born around 1313.[8]

Robert Raymes, born in *c.* 1301/04, a former sheriff of Northumberland who lived in Aydon near Hexham, a few miles west of Newcastle-upon-Tyne, died on 10 October 1349. His widow Agnes married a second husband, Robert Louther, and died in October 1362, and Agnes's son from her first marriage, Nicholas Raymes, was born in *c.* 1339 and was about 10 years old when he lost his father. He died in October 1394.[9] Robert Eslyngton, who was about 46 years old and lived near Alnwick about 35 miles north of Newcastle, also died on 10 October 1349, and his son George died just three days later. George must still have been young; his sisters Christiana, Elizabeth and Isabel were about 16, 13 and 11 in 1349. They all grew into adulthood and married.[10]

Agnes Graper of Newcastle-upon-Tyne died on 13 October 1349. She had two married daughters who were about 24 and 23 years old in 1349, Maud Strother and Alice Orde, who survived the pestilence, as did a few other Newcastle residents whom Agnes knew: Robert Angerton, the mayor of Newcastle, John Brome, William Gabbedede, William Blaklambe, Hugh Aukernebbe, John Horner and Richard Carpenter. Agnes Graper was born in *c.* 1306 as the eldest of the three daughters of Richard Emeldon (d. 1333), and her mother, or perhaps stepmother, was Christine, who outlived her by fifteen years. Richard Emeldon had served as mayor of Newcastle between about 1309 and 1315, when Agnes was a child, and her son-in-law William Strother also became mayor of Newcastle in 1354, 1356 and 1360. Peter Graper, a relative of Agnes's husband Adam Graper, was yet another mayor of Newcastle.

Agnes's sisters were Maud Emeldon, who was three or four years her junior, and Jacoba Emeldon, who was much younger and was perhaps Agnes's half-sister, born in Newcastle on 23 March 1325, by which time Agnes was already married to Adam Graper (born *c.* 1296). Adam was with his father-in-law Richard Emeldon in London when news came to them on 30 March 1325 of Jacoba's birth, the messenger having taken a week to travel the 280 miles from Newcastle. Jacoba's given name was so unusual – all but unique in fourteenth-century England – that one of the jurors at her proof of age in 1340 expressed his surprise that she had been given 'a man's name'. Jacoba was married to Alan Claverying by March 1342, and by early 1365 had wed her second husband John Strivelyn, which means 'Stirling', and he was indeed born in Scotland. She died in 1391 in her 60s. Agnes Graper's other sister Maud also married twice, as did Agnes's younger daughter Alice Orde née Graper and Agnes's mother or stepmother Christine.[11]

John Musgrave was born in Heaton, Northumberland (now a suburb of Newcastle-upon-Tyne) on 14 February 1345, son of John Musgrave the elder and Margaret Ryhill or Ryal. John's maternal grandfather Robert Ryhill died in February 1362, having outlived his daughter and son-in-law by many years. John Musgrave's proof of age was taken in Newcastle in August 1367, and the jurors were all men who had survived the pestilence of 1349 as adults;

they included Edmund Craucestre, born *c.* 1307, John Killingworth, born *c.* 1321, Richard Horsley, born *c.* 1325, who had a son William born in 1345, and Nicholas Houghton, born *c.* 1327, who had a son Geoffrey also born in 1345. Richard Cramelyngton, born *c.* 1327, married his wife Juliana in 1345, and they were both still alive in 1367. John Musgrave, born in 1345, had a son, also John, who died in December 1420, and a grandson Robert, born in *c.* 1390.[12]

Chapter 20

Aftermath

On 26 May 1349, John Bockyng was born in Coddenham, north of Ipswich, and in early November 1349, two couples married in Coddenham: Joan Hauvyll and Roger Eston, and John and Katherine Shyth.[1] Perhaps the four newlyweds were cautiously optimistic that the plague was now over. Another child who came into the world in the terrible year of 1349 was Walter FitzWarin, born in Box, Wiltshire on 15 August, the feast of the Assumption. He was the son and heir of the unusually named Bevis FitzWarin (d. November 1362) and was named after his godfather Walter Pavely. At Walter FitzWarin's proof of age in 1373, all twelve jurors stated that they knew his age and date of birth because they were present in the church during his baptism; 'the church is dedicated to the Assumption, and they were there on that day in one company as pilgrims'. Perhaps they wished to give thanks for surviving the pestilence. Walter FitzWarin inherited a house, arable land, a meadow and woodland in Westbury, north of Warminster.[2] In London, Simon Adyngton's widow Joan gave birth to Simon's posthumous son John at the end of 1349, and by 12 March 1350 had married her second husband, Thomas Neuport. Also in London, Walter Turk, a fishmonger, replaced John Lovekyn as mayor of the city in the annual election held on 28 October every year.[3] In the Cumberland village of Bromfield near Aspatria, 300 miles northwest of London, Thomas Langrigg killed William Tabard, for unstated reasons, on 24 August 1349. Around the same time in Horton, Northamptonshire, William Spicer stabbed his associate William Morflet in the back during a bad quarrel. Spicer fled; Morflet lived long enough to make his final confession and to receive the last rites.[4]

Edward III proclaimed on 1 December 1349 that no-one was allowed to leave England, which was 'much depopulated by the pestilence, and the treasury exhausted'.[5] Ordinary life began, in some ways, to resume, though the population of England was vastly, shockingly smaller than it had been just a few months earlier. Walter Foxcote and Alice Dodyton married in Stepple, Shropshire at Christmas 1349, and a few months later, their neighbour Richard Passeman built himself a new house.[6] John Baskerville, son of Walter Baskerville and Elizabeth Lacy, was born on 10 February 1350 in Lawton in rural Shropshire and was baptised in nearby Diddlebury on the same day. John was born posthumously: Walter Baskerville had died on 24 July 1349, six and a half months earlier, and John's only sibling, Margaret, was born in late November or December 1348, a few months before their father died. The widowed Elizabeth Baskerville née Lacy married a second husband, John Delves, and her son John Baskerville died on 3 April 1374 at the age of 24, leaving a 20-month-old son, also called John. John the father's widow Katherine also married a second husband and outlived her first by half a century, dying in 1423. This Baskerville family were probably not haunted for generations by an enormous hound, but both Walter and his son John died young and did not live to see their children grow up, and little John Baskerville, having lost his father in 1374 when he was a baby, died at the age of 10 on 2 January 1383. Walter's brother Richard Baskerville, however, had descendants.[7]

Joan Modesley gave birth to her son William on 15 August 1350 in the Somerset village of Mudgley, seven miles from Glastonbury. His godparents were William Colne, Simon Michell and Beatrice Bradreney; in the fourteenth century, boys always had two godfathers and a godmother, while girls had two godmothers and a godfather. William Modesley's baptism took place in the church in nearby Wedmore on the same day that John Palmere, recently made a chaplain, celebrated his first Mass there. A crowd of John Palmere's friends and well-wishers were present in the church to support him, and Ralph Barwe and Joan Chiplegh married in Wedmore church that day.[8] In Maidstone, Kent on 19 May 1350, Nicholas Huntyngton proved that he had been born in nearby Yalding on 12 March 1328, and was now old enough take possession of his inheritance from his late father John – who died in the pestilence on 16 April 1349 – in Yalding. The inheritance included a house, ten acres of pasture for sheep and one and a half acres of meadow. Residents of Yalding who lived through the pestilence included John atte Watere, Anselm Ide, Thomas Godying, and John atte Stokke and his son of the same name, who was a few weeks older than Nicholas Huntyngton.[9]

A few English people decided to travel to the great pilgrim site of Santiago de Compostela at the start of the 1350s: Robert atte Grene from Suffolk departed in March 1351, and Henry Clerk, also from Suffolk and in his early 20s, left in the autumn of that year. Robert Bewmays of Coddenham in Suffolk left England for Santiago sometime in late 1348 or early 1349, and rather remarkably given the timing of his long journey, lived to tell the tale; he was still alive in 1370. People whose finances did not permit the journey to Spain, or who preferred to stay in England, travelled instead to the shrine of Our Lady in Walsingham, Norfolk, or to the shrine of St Thomas Becket in Canterbury Cathedral.[10]

In June 1349, Edward III's government passed the Ordinance of Labourers, which forbade people to ask for wages higher than they had been before the pestilence. The legislation was rushed out so quickly that it seems almost pre-emptive.[11] As early as 18 July 1349, some bakers' assistants in London were indicted by the mayor and sheriffs for trying to charge double or triple their previous wages. They were William Osprenge, Ralph atte Hoke, John Chaumpeneys, William Bergeveny, John Maneys and Martin Mynour. On 12 October, four curriers (people who prepared tanned leather for use in saddles, gloves etc) of London, Roger Codyngton, John Phippe, William Aleger and Thomas Caldecote, were also indicted for 'selling leather at a higher price than formerly'. They tried to charge 3 shillings and 6d for a cowhide that once cost 2 shillings, and 9 shillings for an oxhide that once cost only 5 shillings.[12] Even while the Black Death continued to rage throughout the kingdom, workers were prevented from benefiting from the sudden, drastic shortage of labour.

On a much more heartening note, the London authorities took swift and decisive action against people who tried to take advantage of vulnerable orphans, even before the terrible first pandemic was over. As noted above in Chapter 14, Robert Wodham was forced to return money and items that he had stolen from young Ellen Parmenter, the only survivor of her family, on 7 September 1349. On 26 August 1349, the mayor and sheriffs of London ordered John Cantebrigg, Robert Hyngeston and Simon Chikesond to be imprisoned 'on a charge of withholding from children moneys left to them by their father'. The children in question were Margery and Juliana, daughters of the late John Sellyng, who had left £10 worth of possessions including a set of silver spoons, silver rings and silver cups with his executor Henry

Assshebourn to be given to his daughters when they came of age. Henry also died in the pestilence, and Cantebrigg, Hyngeston and Chikesond were three of Henry's own executors and admitted to unlawfully detaining the Sellyng children's goods. A jury found that Cantebrigg 'still had in his possession sufficient goods belonging to the testator to pay the £10 due to the children', and he was ordered to do so. Henry Asshebourn's two other executors were John Pampesworth and Amy Rokesbourgh, who helped to uncover their fellow executors' theft, and a couple named William and Margery Stokes, acting as the 'next friends of Margery and Juliana' Sellyng, brought the matter to the attention of the authorities.[13] It is worth noting that the three children in question, Ellen Parmenter and Margery and Juliana Sellyng, were all female and, in contrast to later eras, English women of the fourteenth century were able to own and inherit goods, land and money. It is also worth noting that one of Henry Asshebourn's executors, one of the two who acted to protect the Sellyng children's interests, was a woman, Amy Rokesbourgh.

Throughout late 1349 and 1350, arrangements were made to place orphaned children in the custody of guardians. This was by no means easy, and not only because such a large percentage of the population was dead. A nationwide rule implemented throughout the fourteenth century and intended to safeguard children held that they could not be sent to live with relatives 'to whom their inheritance would descend at their death'. Contemporaries recognised the risks inherent in sending children to live with people who would benefit financially if they died. On the other hand, orphans were never placed in the custody of complete strangers. Their guardian had to be someone who could be expected to take a keen interest in their well-being and, if no relative was still alive, their parents' executor might be chosen, or a close family friend, or at the very least someone who was a member of the same guild as the orphans' father.

Agnes Stokwell, the 7-year-old from Whitecross Street in London who lost her parents, her four siblings, her aunt and her uncle in 1349, was placed in the care of her late father Walter's apprentice, Thomas Bournham.[14] Given that Thomas was still an apprentice, it is highly likely that he was under 20 years old and was perhaps as young as 16 or so. He was, however, someone who was known to little Agnes, a familiar face in a world where her entire family had been wiped out in a few months, and was someone who could earn a decent wage and provide for them both. Agnes and Thomas vanish from written record after 1350; one hopes that they lived long and thrived.

Nicholas Werlingworth came from the village of Worlingworth in Suffolk, and forged a successful career as a goldsmith in London. He married a woman named Joan, and Thomas, their only child, was born in or not long before September 1337. The small family lived on Friday Street near St Paul's Cathedral, about a mile from Agnes Stokwell's home in Whitecross Street. Nicholas made his will on 1 May 1349, and died within days. Joan did not remain a widow for long, and died before late August 1349. In her will, she asked to be buried near her husband in St Paul's churchyard, and declared her wish that her late husband's friend John Bret should look after her son Thomas Werlingworth and his inheritance until he came of age. John Bret, however, also died not long before 19 October 1349, leaving Thomas in the care of his wife, another Joan. Joan Bret was, sadly, also ailing and passed away shortly afterwards. Twelve-year-old Thomas was left alone in the world. At an assembly of the mayor and the remaining aldermen of London, it was decided that the boy should live with John Hiltoft, who was another goldsmith and must have been known to Thomas's father. Thankfully, John survived the pestilence and lived until 1368.

Thomas Werlingworth followed in the footsteps of his late father and his guardian and became a goldsmith. After he came of age in 1358, he lived in the house on Friday Street that he had inherited from his parents, and ran a brewery there as well as his successful goldsmithing business. Thomas never married but had a long-term relationship with Christine Ippegrave, who came from another family of goldsmiths, and they had three sons, John, Thomas and William, in the late 1350s and early 1360s. Why the couple did not marry is unclear. In March 1364, Thomas Werlingworth became seriously ill, and died in May 1365, aged 27. He asked to be buried in St Paul's churchyard near his parents, and left his house on Friday Street and everything in it to his partner Christine for the rest of her life. Thomas also gave the three young boys £5 each and left them in Christine's custody. This was a kindness both to her and to their sons, as in the fourteenth century it was not always a given that a mother would be appointed as her children's guardian, especially when they were born outside marriage. By April 1370, John the eldest Werlingworth/Ippegrave son had died, and Christine had married a man named William Thaksted.[15]

Thomas Wychard of Congerstone in Leicestershire died around 1 August 1349 when his son John was 6 years old, and John, who had already lost his mother as well, was sent to live with his maternal grandfather Edmund Appelby. Edmund probably lived in the village of Appleby Magna, six miles from Congerstone, and would not receive John's small inheritance from his father if anything happened to the boy. He was also someone who could be expected to take good care of his late daughter's child, and evidently did so: John Wychard lived until 1405, and died in his early 60s.[16]

The draper Thomas Canterbury and his wife Margery both died not long before 12 March 1349, and their young sons John, Simon, William and Thomas were suddenly orphaned. The boys had an older half-brother, Thomas Kent, Margery's son from a previous marriage, who was already an adult earning a wage and assumed responsibility for them.[17] Katherine, widow of another draper, Thomas Holebech, made her will on 26 March 1349 and died before 4 May that year. She left her children Bartholomew, William and Alice, and the apprentices she was teaching, in the custody of her father John Pecche, though Bartholomew Holebech, still alive when Katherine made her will, died before 6 May 1350.[18]

Ten-year-old William Burdeyn lost his father Walter, a London goldsmith, to the pestilence, and a guardian, Thomas atte Barnet, was appointed for him at the end of July 1349. Thomas lost his own father John atte Barnet in or before late 1349, and was probably only a young adult when he assumed responsibility for young Walter, as his brother Roger was under 21 when their father made his will in March 1349. By the late 1360s, Thomas atte Barnet was a master stonemason and had married a woman called Katherine. He was still alive in 1377, though, sadly, his and Katherine's children all died young. William Burdeyn himself became a goldsmith like his late father and was still alive in 1383, aged 44.[19] The three sons of Hugh Plastrer – Robert, aged 12, John aged 9 and Thomas, aged 6 – were orphaned in April 1349 and given into the custody of William Oyldebeof (which means 'Bull's Eye') of Colmworth in Bedfordshire.[20] The relationship between William and the three Plastrer brothers is not stated, but he was perhaps their maternal uncle, or a close friend of their late father.

Tragically, the Black Death, whatever people might have believed in late 1349, had not gone away. King Alfonso XI of Castile-León died of the plague in late March 1350, a very high-profile victim. His 15-year-old son Infante

Pedro succeeded him, and had Edward III's daughter Joan of Woodstock not herself fallen victim to the plague in the summer of 1348, she would now have become queen consort of Castile-León. Back in England, the sisters Joan and Elizabeth Walsh, whose cousin Elizabeth Salmon née Seyncler had died in Chickerell, Dorset on 10 October 1348, died a few hours apart on the same day, 10 August 1350. Joan died first, around sunset, and Elizabeth followed at around midnight. In June 1339, several months after their father Nicholas Walsh died, Joan was said to be 2 years old and Elizabeth 1, so when they died, they were about 13 and 12. They were survived by their aunts Alice and Joan Walsh, their cousin Simon Brit, their cousin Elizabeth's son John Salmon and Elizabeth's younger sisters Joan, Lucy and Christine Seyncler.[21] And the pestilence would return to England again and again over the next few years and decades. The horror was not yet over.

Part II

The Later Pandemics

Chapter 21

The Second Pandemic, 1361/62 (1)

The year 1361 was an odd one, which saw – in stark contrast to the awful summer of 1348 – a drought in England and northern France, and around late May that year, before the long dry spell began, a rain 'almost like blood' fell. People claimed to have seen apparitions in the sky, including a cross made of blood, and in England, France and other countries, supposedly two castles appeared in the air from whence two armies of men, one dressed in black clothes and the other in white, sallied forth and did battle before vanishing again. It was a year of strange wonders and signs, and the pestilence came back in full force after an absence of eleven years. The *Brut* chronicle, written in Middle English, states that the second pandemic of 1361/62 was 'a great and huge pestilence of people' that affected men more than women, and that widows, 'as women out of governance', coupled with and married men 'that were of low degree [status] and little reputation'. The *Anonimalle* chronicle, written in England in medieval French, says that the second pandemic of the early 1360s was called 'the mortality of children' (*la mortalite des enfauntz*) and that a great number of children died and were 'commanded to God'. Nor did matters improve much as 1362 came round: a terribly destructive storm swept across England and elsewhere in northern Europe in January that year. As keen as ever to prevent workers benefiting in any way from natural disasters, Edward III and his government ordered the mayor of London not to allow tilers in the city to increase the price of tiles 'by pretext of the damage done by the recent tempest'.[1]

King Edward and Philippa of Hainault's youngest daughters Mary of Waltham, born in October 1344, and Margaret of Windsor, born in July 1346, both died not long after 1 October 1361. Given the timing, it seems likely that they fell victim to the second pandemic as their sister Joan of Woodstock (born *c.* January 1334) had fallen victim to the first one. Margaret's death left John Hastings, heir to his late father Laurence's earldom of Pembroke, a widower at just 14 years old. He later married Anne

Manny, whose Hainaulter father Walter Manny had established a cemetery for plague victims near London. Another royal kinsman who perhaps died in the second pandemic was Henry of Grosmont, first duke of Lancaster and earl of Leicester, Lincoln and Derby. He died on 23 March 1361 in his town of Leicester, in his late 40s or early 50s.

In Earl's Colne in Essex, Maud Ufford, the 16-year-old countess of Oxford, was pregnant in 1361 with her only child, Robert de Vere, who was born on 9 January 1362 and named after his great-uncle and godfather Robert Ufford, earl of Suffolk (d. 1369). Robert de Vere, earl of Oxford, would grow up to become the notorious favourite and perhaps lover of Edward III's grandson and successor Richard II. His other godfather was Simon Sudbury, elected bishop of London in 1361 and archbishop of Canterbury in 1375, who would be murdered in London during the Peasants' Revolt in 1381.[2] Sudbury's predecessor as bishop of London, Michael Northburgh, died at Copford in Essex on 9 September 1361, apparently of plague. In his will, Michael referred to himself as an 'unworthy minister of the Church in London' and, among his numerous bequests, he ordered the huge sum of 1,000 marks (£666.66, well over a million pounds in modern terms) 'to be placed in a chest to stand in the treasury of St Paul's' to provide loans for those who needed one. He also gave £100 to 'poor scholars of canon and civil law' at Oxford.[3]

On Monday, 5 July 1361, John Kilryngton and Alice Laumprey married in Ashford, Devon, and on the same day in the same place, Joan Grede married John Holm. Cousins Richard Gamboun and Philip Gamboun were both born in Ashford in the summer of 1361.[4] Elizabeth Staunton was born in Thornhill, Yorkshire on 12 March 1361 and named after her godmother Elizabeth Roklay. She lost her father William when she was very young and her grandfather Geoffrey Staunton, born in *c.* 1302, in 1370.[5] Three residents of Whitchurch in Shropshire, Hugh Lewys, Robert Brere and John Erdeston, were attacked and robbed in nearby Marbury on 22 June 1361, while William Mineton and Thomas Whitchurche, also from Whitchurch and both in their early 30s, set off together on pilgrimage to the Holy Land three days later on 25 June. Despite the second pandemic and the dangers of the long journey, they both returned home safely and were alive in the 1380s. A tragic accident occurred in the Northamptonshire village of Great Doddington when 4-year-old Joan and 3-year-old Margaret, daughters of

Thomas and Agnes Aleyn, accidentally started a fire that soon burned out of control while they were trying to heat a brass dish. Both little girls perished.[6]

The king pardoned Thomas Stace in February 1361 for raping Cecily Pypere and abducting Isabel Parkeman in 1359, and for subsequently escaping from prison in Canterbury. In April 1361, Alice Almand was found to have killed John Langetoft, a chaplain, in self-defence, and was subsequently released from Newgate prison in London. Thomas Crispyn, a one-man crime wave from Grimsby in Lincolnshire, received a royal pardon for numerous crimes also in April 1361, thanks to his 'good service in the war against France'. His dozens of crimes included beating up Walter White, Adam Spenser and William Sywan, setting fire to Nicholas Hustwayt's house in Burton-upon-Stather while Nicholas was inside, stealing a silver cup from Emma Wytheryn's house in Bradley near Grimsby, stealing Thomas atte Wode of Grimsby's horse, stealing two barrels of herring from a ship at Humberston and breaking numerous men out of prison. And the king took a keen interest in the welfare of Richard Wolf of Barnstaple in Devon, whose father Walter died in the summer of 1352 when Richard was a baby. It transpired that the prior of Pilton Abbey near Barnstaple had married 10-year-old Richard off to his 12-year-old illegitimate daughter Denise, whom he had fathered while a monk at Malmesbury Abbey in Wiltshire. As Denise was below Richard in rank, their marriage was considered to disparage him, which was contrary to the Statute of Merton of 1236. Edward III therefore sent men to take custody of Richard until it was decided what should be done about his marriage.[7]

There was a John Pavely who was born near Northampton in July 1333 and succeeded to his family's lands in the Midlands when his three older brothers died in the summer of 1349 (see Chapter 11 above). Another man named John Pavely came from Westbury in Wiltshire, and was born around 1305/07. From his first marriage to a woman called Elizabeth, John had a daughter named Alice Pavely. With his second wife Agnes de la Mare, widow of John Forstell, he had another daughter, Joan Pavely, born in Westbury on 14 November 1353. Agnes Pavely née de la Mare died on 5 October 1361; her husband John died on 21 October; and John's daughter Alice from his first marriage died on the same day as her father, a few hours later. Joan Pavely was not yet 8 years old when she lost both her parents and her older half-sister Alice. Joan's mother and maternal uncle Robert de la Mare (born *c.* 1315/18) were the children of Peter de la Mare, who died on 16 August 1349, apparently a victim of the first pandemic. It seems virtually certain that Agnes and her husband and stepdaughter died in the second pandemic. Agnes's daughter Joan Pavely survived and married Ralph Cheyny, with whom she had a son, William Cheyny (*c.* 1374–1421).[8]

In Woodbury in Devon, a few miles from Exeter, William Aumarle died on 15 November 1361, and his 12-year-old son William Aumarle the younger died on 16 April 1362. William the father was born in *c.* 1323 and was about 38 at the time of his death, and in 1347 had become the godfather of Margaret Dinham, great-granddaughter of Margaret Hydon (see Chapter 3 above). His daughters Margaret Aumarle, born in *c.* 1343, and Elizabeth Aumarle, born in *c.* 1345, outlived their younger brother.[9] Another pair of father/son victims in Devon were Nicholas Seymour, who died in North Molton a few miles east of Barnstaple on 13 October 1361, and his elder son, also Nicholas, who was about 9 years old and died on 21 October 1361. The younger Nicholas's 6-year-old brother Richard Seymour survived, though was left an orphan; his mother Muriel was already dead. Richard Seymour was born in Rode, Somerset on 3 September 1355, and named after his godfather Richard, vicar of Frome. One of the jurors who took part in Richard's proof of age in Bruton in September 1376 was Nicholas Cadebury, who had been hired to build a new hall for Joan Chasteleyn's father Thomas in Dinnington in March 1348 (see Chapter 3) and was about 50 in 1376.[10]

Robert Eslyngton and his son George, who lived near Alnwick in Northumberland, died on 10 and 13 October 1349 (see Chapter 19), though Robert's daughters Christiana, Elizabeth and Isabel survived the first pandemic. Elizabeth, the middle Eslyngton daughter, born in *c.* 1336, died shortly before 12 April 1362, and her husband Gilbert Heron died on the same day. Isabel, born *c.* 1338/39, was now the only member of the Eslyngton family still alive.[11]

John Pappeworth (born *c.* 1300) of Papworth St Agnes in Cambridgeshire died on 30 September 1361; his 27-year-old daughter-in-law Elizabeth née Preston, wife of his 30-year-old son William, died on 2 October; and Elizabeth's father John Preston died on 22 September. Elizabeth and William Pappeworth had had a son who died young, and Elizabeth had no siblings. Her heirs were her four living aunts, her father's sisters Eleanor, Margaret, Katherine and Cecily Preston, and her cousins Felicia and John, children of her other two aunts Alice and Christine Preston. Her widower William Pappeworth died in September 1414 in his 80s, having married a second wife, Alice.[12] In the Buckinghamshire village of Marsh Gibbon, Thomas atte Pole died on 24 October 1361, and his daughter Katherine, just 1 month old at the time, survived him by only a few months and died on 6 June 1362.[13]

John Beauchamp was born on 20 January 1330 in Stoke-sub-Hamdon in Somerset, six miles from Hinton Saint George, and died on 29 September 1361 'immediately before sunset'. His mother Margaret St John died on either 6 or 21 November 1361. John's widow Alice, whose maiden name was also Beauchamp, lived for another twenty-two years. John's older sister Cecily outlived him by decades as well, and their nephew John Meriet, born on 24 March 1346 as the son of their other sister Eleanor Beauchamp, lived through all the pandemics of the Black Death.[14] Also in Stoke-sub-Hamdon, Robert Latimer died on either 28 August or 4 September 1361, and his widow Katherine died on 2 November. Katherine had a 12-year-old son, William, from her previous marriage to Andrew Turbervill, while her son with her second husband, also called Robert Latimer, was, heartbreakingly, just a baby when he lost both his parents: he was born on 22 May 1361 in Dewlish, Dorset. The little boy's older half-brother William Turbervill also died young at an uncertain date, perhaps in 1361. Robert Latimer the elder had been in good enough health a few months before his death to be summoned to attend a parliament held at Westminster in January/February 1361. He was born in *c.* 1316, so was in his mid-40s when he died, and his wife Katherine, given that she was still young enough to give birth in 1361, was probably under 40. Their son Robert Latimer the younger was alive in 1412, and had recently married his second wife, Maud Hulle. Someone, presumably a surviving relative, took good care of him, and to remove the infant from the house where both his parents had died of the pestilence took considerable courage and compassion on someone's part.[15] Another Katherine Latimer died in Leicestershire on 9 August 1361. She was the widow of Warin Latimer aka Latimer Bochard of Braybrooke (see Chapter 12), who had died in August 1349.[16]

William Hadresham of Coombe near Kingston-upon-Thames in Surrey, born in the mid or late 1320s as the son of Nicholaa Nevill of Blaxwell in Wiltshire and John Hadresham, died shortly before 1 September 1361. His son John was only a few months old, born on 13 December 1360.

As there is no record of William's wife alive after 1361, it appears that their son was, like Robert Latimer, orphaned as a baby, and that he was raised by his father's younger brother John, who was also his godfather. In 1368, the manor-house of Coombe that was part of the young John's inheritance from his father and grandparents 'was by some of his servants accidentally burnt'. John Hadresham died on 28 October 1417 a few weeks before turning 57, and his wife Agnes was pregnant at the time. There is no record of a child, however, so either Agnes miscarried, or the child was stillborn or died very young. John was outlived by his cousins Alice Virly and Joan Silverton, daughters of William Hadresham's sister Christine.[17]

The Nevill Family of Wiltshire and Hadreshams of Surrey

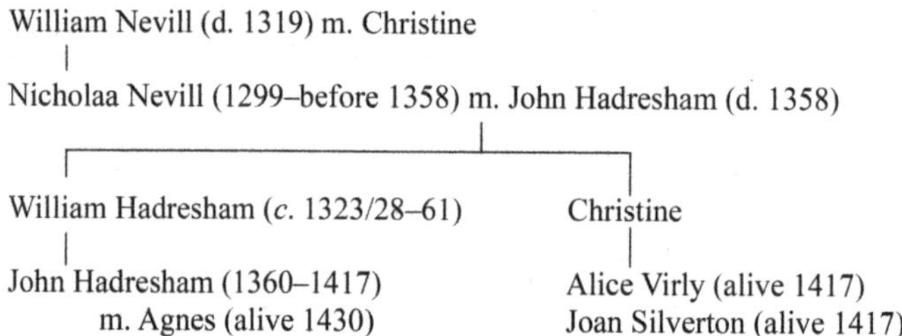

In Comberton in Cambridgeshire, Maud Burdeleys died on 3 August 1361, and her sister-in-law Elizabeth Burdeleys, widow of Thomas Mareschal, died on 10 September 1361. Maud's late husband John Burdeleys, Elizabeth's brother, was born in *c.* 1327 and died in 1347 before he came of age, and Elizabeth was a few years older than her brother, born in *c.* 1319 and in her early 40s when she died. Her sister Joan (born *c.* 1322) had four sons and two daughters with her first husband Gilbert Chambre, and one daughter, Isolda, born in *c.* 1359/60, with her second, John Middleton aka John FitzJohn. Before Joan Chambre née Burdeleys married John Middleton in 1359, she set several conditions for him to fulfil. One, that John should arrange a marriage for her eldest son Edmund Chambre (*c.* 1347/49–1400) with 'a wife of reasonable age having £20 yearly of land and rent at least' before Edmund reached the age of 24; two, that he should pay the debts of her late husband Gilbert and pay for a man to travel to the Holy Land to pray there for Gilbert's soul; and three, that he should provide clothing, food and all other necessaries for her younger Chambre children, Gilbert,

Ellis, Thomas, Margaret and Joan, until they were married. As it turned out, John Middleton 'refused to perform any of the conditions and drove the said children from his house within a year of the marriage'. Joan died in early 1375 and, two and a half years later, her widower (d. 1393) performed the 'office of chief lardener' at the coronation of 10-year-old Richard II, as his wife's great-grandfather Geoffrey Burdeleys had done at the coronation of 14-year-old Edward III in 1327.[18]

John Inkepenne of Woolston in Hampshire (now a suburb of Southampton) died on 24 August 1361, leaving two small sons from his marriage to Isabel. John, the elder, was 3 years old, and Robert, the younger, was born on 1 April 1360 in Winchester and was less than 18 months old when he lost his father. John the elder son died in 1374 perhaps in the fourth pandemic of the Black Death, aged about 16, and his mother Isabel outlived him by many years and died in October 1410, just under half a century after she lost her husband. As well as his and Isabel's two sons, John Inkepenne had an illegitimate son called John Ryver, who was still alive in 1389.[19] Walter Harwedon, a horse dealer of London, made a will on 28 June 1361 and died before 20 July. He was married to a second wife, Marion, and had children Richard, Alice and Joan, one or two of whom were perhaps the children of his first wife, Felicia. By 1368 when she was still only 8 years old, Joan Harwedon, the youngest child, had lost both her parents and her older siblings, though her father's brother William was alive and became her guardian. In or not long before October 1376 at the age of 16, Joan married a goldsmith named Thomas Essex, possibly the person of this name who was the son of Richard Essex, a draper who came originally from Sible Hedingham near Braintree in Essex and moved into London. Richard made his will on the same day as Walter Harwedon and died at about the same time.[20] William of Derby, a tailor, made his will on 5 June 1361, and both he and his wife Agnes's son Edmund were already dead when Agnes made her will a week later. She died either on 15 June or a day or two later. Agnes and William had a daughter, Edmund's younger half-sister Alice Outpenne, who made her will on 1 July and died soon afterwards, and suddenly a whole family was gone within barely a month. Agnes left bequests in her will to John Sulby, a relative, but John died before 20 July 1361 while his wife Edith was pregnant.[21]

Richard of Wycombe, a corder (maker of cord) in London, died shortly before 10 May 1361, leaving a widow, Pernel, and daughters Alice, Joan and Isabella. Alice and Joan, who was a nun of Barking Abbey, were probably born to Richard's first wife Christine, while Isabella was Pernel's daughter. Born in early 1352, she was only 9 when she lost her father, and her mother and her half-sister Alice also died before 4 July 1361, when Isabella was given into the custody of a man named William Grenyngham. Her nearest living relative in the secular world was now her cousin John, son of one of her father's three brothers. Richard of Wycombe left Isabella 200 marks (£133.33) of silver as her dowry and his 'best silver *spicedysshe*' (spice-dish), and the temptation of such a large marriage portion proved too great for someone: within weeks of her father's death, Isabella was 'carried off and could not be found'. Horribly, it transpired during an investigation seven years later that the child had died not long after her abduction, perhaps from the plague or perhaps from the trauma of losing her family and then being kidnapped.[22]

Chapter 22

The Second Pandemic, 1361/62 (2)

Roger and Maud Cifrewast of Clewer near Windsor died on 28 May and 21 June 1361 respectively. Roger was born in 1311 or 1312 so was almost 50 when he died, and his and Maud's son John was about 22 in 1361.[1] Margery St John of Basing (now Old Basing) in Hampshire died on 19 October 1361, and her 3-year-old son John St Philibert died on 13 November. Margery's brother Edmund had died during Edward III's siege of Calais in August 1347 when he was probably only 14 years old. She was a few years Edmund's senior, born in *c.* 1329 and about 32 when she died in the second pandemic.[2] In Great Givendale near Pocklington in Yorkshire, where the Arblaster family (see Chapter 18) came from, John Stra died on 30 December 1361, and was survived by his sisters Isabel Stra, aged 22, and Joan Stra, aged 20. The siblings' late father, William Stra, was born around 1312 and died in 1350.[3]

Katherine Clifton of Little Waltham near Chelmsford in Essex died on either 14 or 28 December, and Alice Chambre of Weston-sub-Edge in Gloucestershire died on the 9th. Katherine's husband Constantine Clifton must have died at the same time that she did, though the date of his death is not recorded. They left a son who was just 8 years old, John Clifton, born in Little Waltham on 15 August 1353. Alice Chambre, who had no children, had been one of five sisters, and was outlived by the eldest, Sibyl Pope. Her other three sisters, Katherine Acton, Agnes Bentham and Margery Solers, were already dead.[4] John Giffard of Weston-sub-Edge, who was born in October 1327 and proved his age in October 1348 (see Chapter 5 above), died in November 1356 when his only child, Elizabeth, was 4 years old. Elizabeth Giffard died on 3 November 1361 at the age of 9, perhaps a victim of the second pandemic. The manor-house called Giffard's Manor passed to her father's cousin, also John Giffard.[5]

Joan Daubeney of Kingsholm in Gloucestershire died on 20 September 1361, and her husband Richard died on 29 September. They must have been a young couple: Richard's sister Elizabeth Daubeney was not yet 7 years old in September 1361, having been born in Cromhall, Gloucestershire on 11 November 1354. Richard and Elizabeth's father Ellis or Elias Daubeney (born *c.* 29 September 1315) outlived his son by more than twenty years and died in February 1384. By June 1369, when she was 14, Elizabeth Daubeney was married to Gilbert Giffard, and later married a second husband, Andrew Wauton.[6] In June 1387, Andrew was murdered by a chaplain, Robert Blake, and another man, John Ball, at his wife's instigation. Elizabeth Wauton née Daubeney was burned alive in April 1388, the customary – though thankfully very rare – punishment in the fourteenth century for women who killed their husbands (see also the fate of Alice Wake in Chapter 3 above). John Ball was drawn, hanged and quartered for the murder, while Robert Blake, as a chaplain, was handed over to the ecclesiastical authorities to deal with.[7]

Thomas Mynstede died on 25 September 1361 in Minstead, a village in the New Forest in Hampshire. He and his wife Sybil had two daughters: the elder was apparently called Juliana, though in one record is named as Isabel, and the younger was Christine. Juliana was born on 1 May 1357 and Christine on 1 August 1358. The sisters were heirs to their father's house, nine acres of arable land, an acre of meadow and forty acres of woodland, and were still alive in the early 1380s, as was their mother, Sybil.[8] Another New Forest victim was 12-year-old Thomas Reyson of Upper Burgate, who died on 20 August 1361.[9] In Burnham in Buckinghamshire, John Huntercombe died on 18 May 1349 during the first pandemic, and his widow Christine died on 20 or 21 October 1361 during the second. John was probably born in 1304 so was in his mid-40s when he died, and he and Christine had a son whose name was also John, born around 1331/34. Christine married a second husband called Nicholas Aumberden in or before November 1350.[10]

Edmund Croupes of Whittington in Gloucestershire was born in *c.* 1332 and died on 24 September 1361. He had an older sister, Alice, who in 1361 was married to Thomas Baskerville, the first of her three husbands, and by 1375 was married to her third, William Barndhurst. She died in 1404 in her mid-70s. Edmund and Alice's father Richard Croupes, who died in 1336 when they were young children, was of illegitimate birth.[11] Robert Danvers of Oxenwood in Berkshire died on 25 September 1361, and his uncle Richard Danvers of Boarhunt Herbelyn in Hampshire died on 13 October 1361. Robert's son Edmund, born in *c.* 1345 and about 16 at the time, survived, and 'departed to parts beyond seas' in 1366. Possibly he took part in the military campaign in Spain that the prince of Wales undertook in 1366/67 to aid King Pedro of Castile-León against Pedro's illegitimate half-brother and deadly enemy Enrique of Trastámara. Edmund Danvers was dead by March 1370.[12] John Ernys of Godshill on the Isle of Wight died on 26 August 1361, and his maternal uncle Thomas Bere, who was in his 40s and lived in Hampshire, died around noon on 22 September. John left two small daughters, 3-year-old Joan and 1-year-old Christine.[13]

William FitzWarin of Wantage in Berkshire died on 28 October 1361, survived by his wife Amice Haddon and their son Ivo, born in Blunsdon St Andrew in Wiltshire on 30 November 1347. Ivo died in September 1414 a few weeks before turning 67.[14] Roger Norman of Kemble in Wiltshire (now in Gloucestershire) died on 5 April 1349, his son Roger the younger, who lived 135 miles away in Cavendish in Suffolk, died on 5 October 1349, and Roger the younger's only child, Giles Norman, died on 21 October 1361 at the age of about 17, leaving a widow named Joan.[15] In London, a mercer named John Stable made his will on 12 December 1361 and died either that day or the following day. His will mentioned his sons William and Thomas and his daughter Isabella, and the child with whom his wife Joan was pregnant. By October 1363, William Stable was dead, as were John's widow Joan and the child born after John's death. Thomas Stable was 4 years old in 1363 and his sister Isabella was 3.[16]

In the Kent hamlet of Leaveland, twelve miles from Canterbury, Thomas Northwode, who was about 27, died on 6 August 1361, and his brother Richard, who was about 22, made his will on 4 September and died on the 30th of that month. Their sisters Joan Lovedale, who came between Thomas and Richard in the birth order, and Agnes Northwode, the youngest child, survived. The four siblings came from a large family: their great-grandfather John Northwode (died before 1319) had nine sons, of whom the fourth eldest, Simon, was the siblings' paternal grandfather. The siblings' father was Simon's son Robert Northwode, who was born in Binbury, Kent in May 1314 and was about 20 when his eldest child Thomas was born in *c.* 1334, and died in July 1360. Robert's youngest child Agnes Northwode was still alive in 1414, a century after her father's birth, and apparently never married.[17]

Another set of brothers who both died during the 1361 pandemic were the Overtons of Wiltshire: Thomas Overton died on 6 September and William Overton on 13 October. They were probably both in their early or mid-40s. William had a 19-year-old son also named Thomas, born in Bishop's Sutton near Alresford in Hampshire on 7 July 1342, and a daughter Isabel (d. 1400), several years younger than her brother. The younger Thomas Overton died on 24 August 1370, aged 28, when his wife Joan was about seven months pregnant with their son Michael.[18] The Overtons lived in the Wiltshire hamlet of Eastcott, then called Escote or Estcote, and another person who died during the 1361 pandemic was Katherine Escote. She was the third and youngest daughter of Eugenia and Adam Bukesgate (d. 1333) and was born on *c.* 2 February 1312. Katherine married Giles Escote and gave birth to her son William in West Tytherley, Hampshire on 26 May 1353, when she was 41 years old. She died on 14 October 1361. Her son William Escote was still alive in May 1404, when he was one of the jurors at Edmund Holland's proof of age. Edmund was heir to the earldom of Kent and a half-nephew of Richard II, and William was present at his baptism in Brockenhurst in the New Forest in early 1383.[19]

John Ore of Guestling, five miles from Hastings in Sussex, died on 7 October 1361, and his 24-year-old son Richard died on 1 November. Richard had one child, a daughter named Amice, who was about a year old when she lost her father and grandfather.[20] John Ryvere of Westrop near Corsham in Wiltshire died on 8 September, his mother Joan died on 3 October and his younger brother Richard, who was in his early 30s, died on 4 December. Richard Ryvere left a widow, Emma (d. 1368), with whom he had a 9-year-old son called Thomas and a 4-year-old daughter called Agnes, who later became a nun at Shaftesbury Abbey in Dorset.[21]

Richard Lacer of Bromley in Kent made his will on Tuesday, 27 July 1361, and died that day or on Wednesday; his wife Isabella made her own will on Thursday, 29 July, by which time she was already a widow. Isabella had a son called William Randolph from a previous marriage, who was still alive and 'of increasing age' at the end of the 1390s, and Richard had a son also from a previous marriage and also named Richard. He left the boy in Isabella's custody, though as Isabella only outlived her husband by a day or two, alternative arrangements must have been made. Richard and Isabella Lacer were buried in the parish church of Bromley.[22] In the port of Sandwich, also in Kent, Thomas atte Welle turned 14 on 3 June 1361, and lost both his mother Agnes and his 18-year-old brother William that year.[23] Osbert Wynter, a poulterer of London, made his will on 25 March 1361 and died before 25 October. He and his wife Mabel had two sons, Thomas, who was 6, and Henry, who was just a year old. In his will, Osbert left custody of the children to Mabel, but she must also have died in 1361, as the little boys were assigned to other guardians.[24]

Robert Guldeford (i.e., Guildford in Surrey), a draper, made his will on 12 May 1361 and died before 27 May, and his widow Joan died shortly before 6 December 1361. Robert and Joan's younger two daughters, Maud and Margery, died as well. Their other children, 11-year-old Rose and 9-year-old Henry, survived, and in his will, Robert specified that his wife should be their guardian after he died. In the end, a few days after Joan died, Rose was sent to live with John Utlicote, a draper like her father, and her little brother was placed with Thomas Kendale, rector of the church of St Augustine near St Paul's in London.[25] Another likely victim of the 1361 pandemic was John Malweyn, who died probably in Pledgdon in Essex on 23 June, two days after he made his will. His daughter Margery had married Nicholas Mockyng of Tottenham (see Chapter 7 above) when they were children in or before 1347, and his heir was his son John Malweyn the younger, who was 17 or 18 in 1361. Margery Malweyn had been widowed from Nicholas Mockyng a few months earlier, and in his will her father forbade her to marry 'a certain John Dovy, mercer, on pain of losing her legacy' of £200.[26]

John atte Marche of Bromham in Bedfordshire, who was about 14 years old, died on 29 August 1361. He had no siblings, but his late father Geoffrey had a brother, Stephen, who was also dead and left a daughter named Alice, John's cousin and nearest living relative. Alice atte Marche, who was a little older than John, was still alive in 1403.[27] Thomas Saffrey of Great Houghton in Northamptonshire, born in *c.* 1316 as the second son of Margery Stane and William Saffrey, who lost his older brother Brian in the first pandemic (see Chapter 11 above), died on 3 or 5 October 1361, apparently a victim of the second pandemic. His younger sister Joan Saffrey survived. In her early 40s in 1361, Joan used the name of her father and older brothers and appears not to have married.[28] John Maunsel of Hempstead in Norfolk died on 6 August 1361 and was outlived by his brother Walter, about 30 years old, who had leprosy and died three years later. John and Walter had nieces called Beatrice Billing and Rose Robell, daughters of their sisters Alice and Mariote. Rose died in 1415 at the age of about 70, having outlived her husband Robert Robell of Great Yarmouth and their son Thomas.[29]

Geoffrey Botiller was a draper in London who was originally called Geoffrey Cutyngdone (i.e., his native Coddington in Nottinghamshire) and changed his name to that of the master draper who taught him his trade, James Botiller. Geoffrey made his will in December 1348 and died before 4 May 1349. His associate and friend William Macchyng from Essex, also a draper, made his will on 22 May 1349 at the height of the first pandemic, though did not die until shortly before 22 November 1361, during the second. William had become well-off in London, and in his will left money to 'six of the poorest of his family' in the village of Matching in Epping Forest, where he grew up. William Macchyng's son John was Geoffrey Botiller né Cutyngdone's godson. In his will of late 1348, Geoffrey left a tenement to his daughter Katherine that would pass to his son John Botiller if she died and then to his godson John Macchyng if both his children died. They did, leaving no children of their own, and John Macchyng also died not long after his father in 1361. John's sisters, William's daughters Christine and Isabella Macchyng, must also have perished. The two Botiller siblings Katherine and John were the last of their family, and John Macchyng's nearest living relative at the time of his death in 1361 was John Wryghte (born *c.* 1358), grandson of William Macchyng's sister Mabel, who duly inherited Geoffrey Botiller's tenement when he came of age. Geoffrey Botiller and William Macchyng had known each other since as far back as the early 1310s, when they first arrived in London at age 12 or 13 and began their apprenticeships with the master draper James Botiller (d. 1318). Now they and all their families, with the sole exception of William's infant great-nephew John Wryghte, were dead in two terrible pandemics of the Black Death.[30]

Chapter 23

The Third Pandemic, 1368/69

A third pandemic of the Black Death, a 'great pestilence of men and of great beasts', struck England in the late 1360s.[1] Richard Holewelle of Ipswich made his will on 29 October 1368, 'seeing the peril of this world and especially of this existing plague'. He died before 26 February 1369, when his will was proved.[2] Roger Watford, a servant of Edward III's eldest daughter Isabella of Woodstock, died 'in the manner of plague' in Watford on 10 September 1368.[3] The death toll in the late 1360s was seemingly nowhere near as high as in the first two pandemics, however, and an inquisition taken in Sussex in 1377 not long after the fourth pandemic of 1374/75 refers to the 'middle pestilence' of 1361/62, i.e., the jurors ignored the 1369 outbreak and held the pestilence of 1374/75 as the third outbreak.[4]

Elizabeth Daubeney of Gloucestershire, who could not possibly have known that she would be burned alive nineteen years later for murdering her second husband Andrew Wauton (see Chapter 22 above), proved in Wotton-under-Edge on 3 July 1369 that she was now 14 years old. A day later and 160 miles away in Sittingbourne, Kent, Thomas Lapyn, son of James (d. 1359) and Juliana, proved that he was born in Murston, now a suburb of Sittingbourne, on 18 October 1347. By the mid-1370s, Thomas had moved to London.[5] At the end of April 1369, in Carlisle in the far north of England, Richard Kirkebride proved that he had been born on 1 February 1346. Richard was just 3 years old when he lost his father, also Richard Kirkebride, at the start of October 1349, and it seems highly likely that the older Richard, who was about 35 at the time, was a victim of the first pandemic. Richard the son died in 1399.[6]

One highly born victim of the 1368/69 pandemic was Thomas Beauchamp, earl of Warwick, who died on 13 November 1369. Born in February 1314 and named after his royal godfather Thomas of Lancaster, earl of Lancaster and Leicester, the earl of Warwick was 55 when he died.[7] John Lovekyn, who served as mayor of London from October 1348 to October 1349, died a year before the earl of Warwick, shortly before 6 November 1368. He was a *stokfisshmongere* by trade, i.e., someone who sold dried unsalted fish, and was survived by his second wife, Margaret. John left money in his will to his first wife Mabel's rather unfortunately named daughter Lettice Gubbe, and also to his apprentice William Walworth, who is known today for being the mayor of London during the Peasants' Revolt of 1381 and for stabbing Wat Tyler to death in front of 14-year-old Richard II.[8] Another likely London victim of the third pandemic was Thomas Gander, a pouch-maker who died shortly before 16 October 1368 and left money in his will to 'each prisoner in *bocardo*'. A *bocardo* meant an argument in scholarly logic from which one could not escape, and in the late Middle Ages was used as a sarcastic word for prison, a place from where one could also not escape.[9]

Joan Oreby, the only child of John and Margaret Oreby, was probably born in May 1351, and was heir to her father, born in West Witton in Yorkshire on Christmas Day 1318. John Oreby, a landowner in Yorkshire and Lincolnshire who also inherited estates in the south of England from his mother Florence, died in early 1354. In or not long before May 1365 in her early teens, his daughter Joan married Henry Percy, the greatest lord in the north of England. Henry was thirty years Joan's senior and was the widower of Mary of Lancaster (d. September 1362), sixth and youngest sister of Henry of Grosmont, duke of Lancaster.[10] Joan Oreby gave birth to her only child, Mary Percy, who was perhaps named in honour of her father's first wife, at Warkworth Castle, Northumberland on 12 March 1368. Lord Percy died on 18 May 1368 and, though his little daughter was just a few weeks old, he left her a valuable book, his 'green primer' (i.e., a prayer-book with a green cover). Joan Oreby, dowager Lady Percy, died on 29 or 30 July 1369 at the age of 18, and her mother Margaret, dowager Lady Oreby, died on 28 August 1369.[11] It seems likely that both women were victims of the third pandemic. Little Mary Percy, not quite 18 months old, had now lost both her parents and all her grandparents, and her much older half-brothers Henry and Thomas Percy – who later became earls of Northumberland and Worcester respectively – must have taken over her care. As a child, she was married to John Southeray, born in the early or mid-1360s as the illegitimate son of Edward III and his mistress Alice Perrers, but, after the king died in

June 1377, Mary's relatives had her marriage annulled and she wed Lord Ros of Helmsley instead.

Richard Salteby of Grantham in Lincolnshire died on 31 July 1369 when his son Thomas was only 3 years old.[12] A London couple named William and Joan Hanhamstede died weeks apart in the spring of 1369, leaving three daughters called Joan, Christine and Margaret, of whom Christine and Margaret were under the age of 16. William's father had died not long before 20 July 1349 in the first pandemic, and William's mother Agnes appears also to have died that year. William became the guardian of his youngest siblings after his parents' deaths and, in 1369, his wife Joan appointed his brother Thomas Hanhamstede as the guardian of their own two underage daughters in her will.[13]

John Longvilers or Longevillers of Tuxford in Nottinghamshire died on 9 March 1361 during the second pandemic of the plague, leaving three small children, of whom two died during the third pandemic. His and his wife Elizabeth's elder son John, who was most probably born in September 1354, died on 30 May 1369 at the age of 14, and John's younger brother Thomas died five days later. Their sister Agnes, born in Haughton in Nottinghamshire on 12 November 1360, just 4 months old when her father died and 8 years old when she lost both of her older brothers, survived. She married Robert Cromwell in or before December 1374.[14]

Thomas Leversete of Shifnal in Shropshire, who was also about 14, died on 17 August 1369, and his mother Joan died on 21 September. His older sisters Alianore and Isolde, aged about 20 and 16, survived. In Greete also in Shropshire, 19-year-old John Halughton, whose grandmother Agnes Halughton died on 10 August 1349 (see Chapter 5 above), died on 15 September 1369. Richard Estham, another Greete resident, died on 8 August.[15] Another young victim was John Rous of Allensmore near Hereford, who died on 31 August 1369, under the age of 21. His heir was his 12-year-old sister Juliana, born on 14 June 1357. The siblings had lost their father Thomas Rous on 6 January 1358 when Juliana was under 7 months old, though their mother Maud was still alive in the 1370s and married to a second husband. Sometime before 3 July 1370, though she was still only 13 years old, Juliana Rous was abducted and forcibly married to one Thomas Hord. Thomas was imprisoned in the Fleet prison in London as a result, and must have died not long afterwards, as Juliana was married to her second husband, Andrew Herle, by June 1374 when she was still only 17.[16]

In the far north of England, in Kirklinton a few miles from Gretna Green, Felicia, widow of Robert Tilliol, died on 17 August 1369. Her son Peter, aged about 13 in 1369, lived until 1435. Felicia's father-in-law, Peter Tilliol the elder (b. *c.* 1299), died on 30 October 1349 during the first pandemic, and was the cousin of John Constable of Holderness in Yorkshire (see Chapter 17 above), who had died a few weeks earlier on 17 September 1349; their mothers Avice and Maud Lascelles were sisters.[17]

William atte Hale of London died in late 1368. He and his wife Agnes had five children: Alice, Mariote, Richard, Thomas and Katherine. The latter two had both joined the Church: Katherine was a nun of the Minoresses' convent off Aldgate near the Tower of London, and Thomas was a canon at Holy Trinity Priory (sometimes called *Cricherche* or Christchurch) also near Aldgate. On 20 November 1368, William atte Hale's will was proved and his widow Agnes was officially appointed as guardian of their children Richard and Alice. Mariote was not mentioned and had perhaps also died. Katherine atte Hale the nun was still alive in October 1387 when her brother Richard, a fishmonger, made his will, and her mother Agnes did not die until 1408, having outlived her first husband William atte Hale by forty years and her second, wine merchant Robert Vanner, by twenty. The atte Hale family owned a building in the Bread Street ward of London called *Boreshede* or 'boar's head', presumably a tavern.[18]

Thomas Poynings, born in Slaugham, Sussex on 19 April 1349 (see Chapter 10), lost his father Michael on 7 March 1369.[19] John Meriet of Somerset, born on 24 March 1346, lost his uncle John Beauchamp during the second pandemic in 1361 (see Chapter 21), then lost his paternal grandmother Isabel on 29 June or 3 July 1369 and his father John Meriet the elder on 2 October 1369. John the elder was born in *c.* late October 1327, so was 18 years old when his son was born in March 1346 and not quite 42 when he died. John Meriet himself survived the third pandemic, perhaps because in 1369 he was overseas 'in furtherance of the war' against the French. When he died in 1391, he left one child, Elizabeth, who despite being only 4 years old was already married to the unusually named Urry Seymour.[20]

Chapter 24

The Fourth Pandemic, 1374/75

The *Anonimalle* chronicle states that the year 1374/75 saw the start of the 'fourth pestilence in many towns in England', especially in the south, and that it subsequently spread to the north. The *Brut* agrees, saying that there was 'a grete pestilens in Engelond' that 'destroyed, violently and strongly, both men and wymmen without noumbre'. Edward III's son John of Gaunt, duke of Lancaster, sent a letter to one of his officials in Yorkshire on 12 October 1375 in which he talked of 'the danger which might arise from this present pestilence'.[1]

William Trumwyn of Cannock died in September 1349 during the first pandemic, and his son William died in November 1361 during the second pandemic, leaving a 7-year-old daughter called Elizabeth and a son called John, then 18 weeks old (see Chapter 13). Eight-year-old John Trumwyn died on 16 October 1369 during the third pandemic. His sister Elizabeth Trumwyn, born in 1354, married Roger Lansant sometime between December 1369 and June 1371, and died childless on 20 July 1375 during the fourth pandemic.[2] It seems likely that the four great pandemics of the Black Death in fourteenth-century England each took a member of the unfortunate Trumwyn family,

On 10 July 1375 in Winchcombe, Gloucestershire, Joan Haym, daughter of the late Richard Haym, proved that she had come of age, and was born in Southam near Cheltenham on 9 August 1357. One of her godmothers was the gloriously named Amflesia Mareschall, and one of the jurors who confirmed her age was John atte Halle, who was about 60 in 1375 and remembered Joan's baptism because the chaplain who performed it 'struck him with a stick and broke his head' on the same day. John failed to explain the reasons for this violent assault by a churchman, though evidently recovered from his injuries. Joan's father Richard Haym died in early December 1361 when Joan was 4, during the second pandemic, though her mother, also named Joan, was still alive in 1393 when an inquisition was held to determine whether she was 'an idiot of unsound mind' (the finding was that she had always been of sound mind and still was). Joan Haym, the daughter, married Richard Lutteleye, her guardian during her minority, between 23 June and 20 October 1375, aged 18.[3]

Four members of the Coggeshale/Baynard family of Essex – see Chapter 14 above – were almost certainly victims of this fourth outbreak of the pestilence. They died on 27 September, 29 September, 8 October and 6 November 1375. An inquisition taken in Cainhoe, Bedfordshire on 12 October 1375 states that ten cottages there had 'newly fallen into the lord [of the manor]'s hands for lack of tenants owing to the pestilence'.[4] Edward Kendale, who owned lands and property in London, Bedfordshire, Hertfordshire and Hampshire, died on 23 or 25 July 1375, aged about 26 or 28; his mother Elizabeth died on 7 or 10 September 1375; and his younger brother Thomas, a clerk who was about 24 or 26, died on 11 or 12 September 1375. Edward and Thomas's sister Beatrice, who had a son and a daughter from her marriage to Robert Turk, survived, as did Edward Kendale's widow, Elizabeth Croiser. The three Kendale siblings must have been born around the time of the first pandemic in the late 1340s, and Beatrice's daughter Joan Turk must have been a mere infant when her two Kendale uncles and her Kendale grandmother died in the fourth pandemic. Beatrice's son, whose name is unknown, died young and perhaps was another victim of the Black Death, and Joan was the heir of the Kendale and Turk families.[5]

The Kendale Family of Bedfordshire

Robert Kendale (d. 1330) m. Margaret (d. 1347)
|
Edward Kendale (*c.* 1309–73) m. Elizabeth (d. 1375)
|
Edward (*c.* 1347/49–75) m. Elizabeth Croiser (d. 1420)
Thomas (*c.* 1349/51–75), a clerk, unmarried
Beatrice (*c.* 1349/51–before 1400) m. Robert Turk (d. 1400)
|
Joan Turk (*c.* 1375–1420) m. John Waleys
|
Beatrice Waleys (b. *c.* 1399) m. Reynold Cokayn
Joan (I) Waleys (b. *c.* 1404) m. Robert Leventhorp
Agnes Waleys (b. *c.* 1411)
Joan (II) Waleys (b. *c.* 1415)

William Olneye, a fishmonger of London who married Isabel Hakeneye in August 1362 (see Chapter 8), made his will on 24 June 1375, and died before 8 September. Isabel, who was 33 in 1375, married her second husband John Wade in or before April 1377, and died in June 1400.[6] Thomas Frowyk of South Mimms in Middlesex (now in Hertfordshire) died not long before 2 April 1375, outlived by his father Henry Frowyk, his wife Maud née Durham, and his and Maud's son, named Henry after his grandfather. Thomas left six oxen, two stallions and 'all his goats' to his father, and his 'two best horses' with their equipment, and five silver goblets and six silver spoons, to his son. Thomas's father-in-law John Durham had died shortly before 29 January 1369 during the third pandemic and was buried in the churchyard of St Giles in South Mimms, and, evidently on good terms with him, Thomas asked to be buried near him, also requesting ten ells of russet cloth and a cross of white cloth to be laid over his dead body. When Henry Frowyk the younger died in February 1386, he requested burial near his father and maternal grandfather.[7]

Edelina Goldburgh was born and raised in Eton near Windsor, and married Thomas atte Legh, a *stokfisshmongere* whose family came from Leatherhead in Surrey and who worked on *Stokfisshmongerrowe* (Stockfishmonger Row) on Thames Street in London. Thomas died in June or July 1373, and Edelina made her will on 27 July 1375 and died before 15 October 1375, perhaps a victim of the fourth pandemic. She and Thomas had no children, and in their wills they both left bequests to various relatives. Thomas's will ended with a very curious and unexplained memorandum 'to restore the value of 40 pence to two men who killed their godfather'. As Thomas Frowyk of South Mimms had, Edelina Goldburgh and Thomas atte Legh both requested that 'a long cloth of russet' with a cross made of white cloth should be laid over their coffins during their funerals, and should afterwards be given to the poor. Among Edelina's numerous charitable requests, she left money to the *Loke* or Lock, a London hospital for lepers founded by Edward II.[8]

Walter Rede, a *wexchaundeller* (wax-chandler) in London, made his will on 21 July 1375 and died before 30 July. He and his wife Gonnora had no children, but Gonnora had a daughter named Agnes from a previous marriage, and Walter requested burial in Agnes's tomb in St Paul's churchyard.[9] Also in or near London, Richard Pembrugge died on 26 July 1375, and his only child Henry, who was 15 or a little younger, died on 1 October 1375. Richard had two older sisters, Amice Burele and Hawise Barre, who were both already dead but left children.[10] Alice Roos or Rous of Radwinter in Essex died on 26 August 1375, and her 13-year-old grandson John Roos died just two weeks later. Alice's son John, young John's father, was already dead, though her daughter Ellen Brokhole lived until August 1419. Young John Roos was already married to a girl called Elizabeth by August 1373, two years before his death, though he was then only 11 years old.[11]

Another young victim in the 1374/75 pandemic was Agnes Sourdevale of Threekingham in Lincolnshire, who died on 6 November 1374 at the age of 11 or 12. Agnes's short life was a rather sad one: she lost her father when she was a baby and her mother when she was about 6, and at Christmas 1372 she was 'seized' by a servant of the prince of Wales in the village of Swine in Holderness, Yorkshire. Despite her youth, Agnes was already married to Alexander Barton at the time of her death, and this marriage was perhaps the intended result of her abduction at Christmas 1372. Agnes was outlived by her paternal grandfather Amand Sourdevale and her great-uncle Thomas, Amand's brother.[12] In Kent, a young aunt and niece died on the same day. Cecily, the 11-year-old daughter of the late Thomas Gravesend, and 16-year-old Joan, daughter of Cecily's late and much older sister (or more probably half-sister) Margaret, both died on 20 July 1375. Their nearest living relatives in 1375 were four second cousins: Alice atte Wode, the brothers John and William Mockyng, and the Mockyngs' younger half-brother Robert Goshalm.[13]

In Much Cowarne near Hereford, Grimbald Pauncefot – who sounds more like a character in the Harry Potter novels than a real person – died on 20 November 1375. Not to be outdone in the fictional-sounding names category, Grimbald's wife was called Pernel Pauncefot.[14] Twenty-five miles south of Much Cowarne, in the tiny settlement of Abenhall in the Forest of Dean, Margaret Abbehale died on 30 September 1375. Born in early April 1341, she was 34 when she died, and was married to her second husband Robert Huntele at the time of her death. Margaret was the daughter of Ralph Abbehale (b. 1317), who died in August 1347 while his wife Isabel was pregnant with Margaret's sister Helen, but the little girl died at just 2 weeks old. Margaret's son John Greyndore, from her first marriage to

Laurence Greyndore, was born in or before November 1358 and died in September 1416.[15]

John Payn died in London on 16 August 1375, and his 3-year-old son William died on 30 September 1375. John's widow Joan was heavily pregnant when she lost her husband and son, and not long afterwards gave birth to her daughter, whose name is recorded as either Emmote (a diminutive of Emma), Amy or Anne. John owned the manor of Vallis near Frome in Somerset as a gift of the Braunche family (see Chapter 3), who held Frome, and presumably he came from that area originally. He was described both as an armourer, i.e., a person who made, sold or repaired weapons, and a *fourbour*, i.e., furbisher, a person who finished or polished bladed weapons. By February 1390, his posthumous daughter was married to Thomas Newton, a mercer.[16] In the village of Skelton near York, 10-year-old Joan Alberton died on *c.* 6 December 1375. Her younger sister Philippa, alive in the summer of 1371, was already dead. Their father Thomas died on 27 July 1369 during the third pandemic, but in 1377 an inquisition wrongly stated that he died, like his elder daughter Joan, during the fourth pandemic in 1375, perhaps representing a confusion as to which outbreak of the Black Death caused Thomas's demise. He was active and apparently hale and hearty in June 1369, the month before he died, implying that his death was sudden. Thomas Alberton's widow Mary, having lost her husband and both of her daughters between 1369 and 1375, married again twice, and died in late 1411 or early 1412. She was, like the late Queen Philippa (d. August 1369), a Hainaulter by birth, and served in the queen's household.[17]

John Mitford, a draper of London, made his will on 31 July 1375, and his son-in-law Henry Padyngton made his own will two days later. Both men died shortly afterwards. Juliana, John's daughter and Henry's wife, survived, and married her second husband Robert Louthe before November 1377. She later married a third, Alexander Walden, and outlived him too. For some reason, Juliana's mother Joan Mitford (d. 1382), John's widow, 'demanded the guardianship' of her grandson John Padyngton, Juliana and Henry's son, 'as his grandmother and next of kin to whom no advantage would accrue at his death'. This was granted, although Henry Padyngton had specified in his will that Juliana should have custody of their son. Henry had also fathered an illegitimate daughter named Katherine atte Pitte with his servant Joan atte Pitte.[18] Another possible London victim was Simon Leggy, whose father

Thomas (d. 1357) had served as mayor of London in 1348 and whose uncle Peter died in 1349 during the first pandemic, and who had a brother also called Simon. He died in or before early November 1375.[19]

Richard Claveryng, another London draper, made his will in August 1375 and died in or before October that year. He requested burial next to his first wife Margaret in St Christopher's church, and had a second wife, Denise. Richard left his goods to his children Alice and Thomas in equal portions, but Alice Claveryng must also have died in 1375. Her brother Thomas, who was about 8 years old, remained in the custody of their mother Denise and her second husband Richard Hatfeld.[20] James Andrew, yet another draper and a former mayor of London, died on 30 September 1374 when his only child Katherine, married to a mercer named John Dovy, was about 19. This is most probably the man of this name whom John Malweyn ordered his daughter Margery in 1361 not to marry (see Chapter 22).[21]

John Weston, a brewer who originally came from St Ives (presumably the one then in Huntingdonshire and now in Cambridgeshire rather than the one in Cornwall) and moved to London, died not long before 17 July 1374. John had embarked with enthusiasm on a marital career, and Margaret, his wife in 1374, was his fourth, following Katherine, the unusually named Joseana and Denise. John had no children of his own, though his fourth wife Margaret had a son and two daughters, and his second wife Joseana had a daughter, all of whom received gifts of cash in John's will. John admitted to having defrauded Geoffrey Taverner, who ran a tavern in Cheapside called the *Bole* ('Bowl'), of 40 shillings or 480d. John's widow Margaret was instructed to restore this amount to Geoffrey in ale, which, given that ale cost only 1d per gallon, would take rather a long time.[22]

In Low Hutton (then called 'Hoton Colswayne') between York and Scarborough, Thomas Bolton died on 20 May 1375, aged about 42. He had one child, Mary Bolton, who was 'aged 2 years less a quarter' on 1 August that year. Thomas's widow Agnes married her second husband John Lokton of Malton near Low Hutton in or before October 1375, and by the early 1390s Mary Bolton had married her stepbrother, William Lokton (d. 1425).[23] John Westlee of Ormesby St Margaret in Norfolk died on 2 October 1374, his wife Burgia Westlee née Ormesby died on 12 October, and Burgia's sister Juliana Fauconer née Ormesby died on 21 October. Neither sister left any surviving children, though Juliana had at least one child with her husband John Fauconer who must have died before her, and Burgia and John Westlee had a son named Thomas who also died before his parents. The sisters' nearest living relatives in the mid-1370s were their cousins Elizabeth Perers, Agnes Snecke and Alice Derlyng.[24] In Langton Wallis in Dorset, a lost medieval village, John Walssh died on 26 October, and his father Roger died four days later. John left a 9-month-old daughter, Joan, and John's sister Margaret Soidon also survived. Joan Walssh married John Fauntleroy before May 1393.[25]

John Estbury of Eastbury in Berkshire died on 26 October 1374; his widow Katherine died on 8 August 1375; and their daughter-in-law Agnes died on 30 June 1375. John and Katherine had three children, who all survived: Agnes's husband John Estbury the younger, who was 29 years old in 1375, Thomas and Edith. Agnes Estbury was just 19 when she died. She was born Agnes Burneby in Watford (a village in Northamptonshire, not the Hertfordshire town of the same name) on 6 May 1356, and married John Estbury the younger sometime before 12 May 1371. Her father Eustace died when she was a small child, and her paternal grandfather Nicholas Burneby of Northamptonshire died on 10 August 1361 during the second pandemic, aged 44, when his elder son Eustace was already dead. Agnes was then 5 years old. She and John Estbury had a child, name and gender not recorded, who died in Agnes's lifetime. John outlived her by more than thirty years and died in August 1406, aged 60, leaving no living children, while Agnes's uncle George Burneby, her father Eustace's younger brother, lived a long life and died in June 1429.

The Burneby/Estbury Family of Berkshire

Eustace Burneby (d. 1343)

Nicholas Burneby (1317–61) m. Alice Astley

Eustace Burneby (d. before 1361) — George Burneby (d. 1429) m. Clemency

Agnes Burneby (1356–75) m. John Estbury (*c.* 1346–1406) — Eustace

Agnes's in-laws the Estburys knew the Wantyng family, who also lived in the village of Eastbury. After John Wantyng died in 1349 during the first pandemic (see Chapter 6 above), his children, William (b. 1337) and Joan, and their property were placed in the custody of John Estbury the elder. In

1372, a few years after William Wantyng died, a house in the village now owned by his sister Joan had its value improved by a dovecot, a windmill and a horse-mill built nearby by John Estbury.[26]

The brothers William and John Stodeye both worked as wine merchants in London, and John served as mayor of London in 1357/58. John made his will on 22 March 1375, though lived through the fourth pandemic and died shortly before 6 September 1376, and William made his own will on 24 August 1375 and was dead by that November. William divided his goods among his wife Isabella, his daughters Katherine and Alianore, and the child with whom Isabella was pregnant at the time of his death. Isabella later gave birth to their third daughter, whom she named Agnes. Agnes Stodeye received £58 as her inheritance from the father she never knew, while her eldest sister Katherine received £133 as dowry from William's estate in August 1376 when she married 18-year-old Richard Brikelesworth, who had been committed to her father's custody in 1371 after his own father died. As many wine merchants did – including Geoffrey Chaucer's father John and uncle Thomas Heyron – William Stodeye lived in Vintry ward, which in modern London is the area near the Southwark Bridge between Blackfriars and Monument. In December 1372, William complained to the Assize of Nuisance that his neighbour Thomas Kynardesle had an extension on his house above the alley leading to William's house but that its roof had fallen in, so that every time it rained water fell on William's land and into his cellar, and was rotting his timbers. By early 1380, his widow Isabella was married to another wine merchant, Philip Derneford.[27]

Another London wine merchant was Roger Longe, who made his will on 29 September 1375 and died shortly afterwards. From his marriage to Lucy, Roger had two legitimate sons named Thomas and William, and also had one illegitimate son, John. He treated all three boys the same in his will. John was about 8 years old when he lost his father, and his legitimate half-brother Thomas was the same age. The other son, William, outlived their father by only a few months. Roger Longe also left money in his will to Maud Beccote or Bectote, presumably a relative, friend, neighbour or servant, 'if she be *enceinte* in the opinion of his executors'. Maud was indeed pregnant, and died soon after giving birth: on 2 August 1376, her daughter Isabel, aged 6 months, was given into the custody of Adam Meryfeld, a goldsmith. Adam was presumably Maud's lover and Isabel's father, though this was not specifically stated. Maud Beccote was not married when Roger Longe made his will, as he left her £20 as her future dowry when she wed and gave her a further 20 marks (3,200d) for her 'uterine child'. After Maud's death, this money was also given into the custody of Adam Meryfeld to look after until little Isabel came of age.[28]

Afterwards

The outbreak of pestilence in the mid-1370s was not the last in medieval England. According to the Westminster Chronicle, a few 'gallant and illustrious' knights died of 'a great and deadly pestilence' during a period of boiling hot weather in England from June to the end of August 1390.[1] It continued to return to England periodically until the famously deadly pandemic of 1665/66.

English literature is enormously richer because some people who were children or young adults in 1348/49 came safely through the first terrible pandemic and subsequent ones, such as Geoffrey Chaucer, William Langland and Julian of Norwich. The *Canterbury Tales* has been so enormously popular for so long that it is hard to imagine a world where it was never written, yet several of Geoffrey Chaucer's close relatives and family associates were taken by the plague, and it is sheer good fortune that he lived through the first two pandemics in 1348/49 and 1361/62 as a child and young adult. Chaucer is believed to have invented, or at least to have been the first person to record, the association of romantic love with St Valentine and his feast day of 14 February. It is curious to imagine that the multibillion-pound Valentine's Day industry might not exist had Chaucer succumbed to the plague before he wrote *The Parliament of Fowls* in the early 1380s.

If John Wycliffe had died of the Black Death in 1349 as a young man at Oxford, the movement of his followers, the Lollards, would not have existed. Wycliffe is considered a significant forerunner to Protestantism and as the 'Morning Star' of the English Reformation, and, if his life had been cut short when he was still a student, the Reformation in this country would surely have developed differently. A boy named Philip Despenser, born in Lincolnshire in October 1342, lost his father Philip Despenser the elder (b. 1313) and his paternal grandmother Margaret Goushill (b. 1294) less than a month apart in the summer of 1349 when he was not yet 7 years old. Philip himself survived the pestilence, married and had children, and his granddaughter and ultimate heir Margery was born at the end of the 1300s. Via her marriage to Roger Wentworth, Margery Despenser was the great-grandmother of Margery Wentworth, mother of Queen Jane Seymour (d. 1537), who became the third wife of Henry VIII in 1536 and the mother of Edward VI (r. 1547–53). If Philip Despenser, a small child when he lost his father and grandmother, had died of the pestilence in 1349, Jane Seymour and her son Edward VI would never have existed. As Edward's short but important reign saw the Reformation in England take great steps forward, if he had never been born because one of his ancestors died of the pestilence as a child, our history would again look very different. Elizabeth Lisle, later Bramshott, born on the Isle of Wight in *c.* 1345, survived all the fourteenth-century pandemics as her father, brother, grandmother, step-grandfather and step-grandfather's son did not, and grew up to have a son who was an ancestor of the Dudley family. If Elizabeth Lisle had died as a child in the plague, Queen Elizabeth I's courtier and favourite Robert Dudley, earl of Leicester, would never have existed; he would not have married Amy Robsart and been suspected of involvement in her mysterious death; he would not have held the great and famous spectacles at Kenilworth Castle in the summer of 1575; and T.S. Eliot would not have made a reference to 'Elizabeth and Leicester/Beating oars' in his 1922 poem 'The Waste Land'.

This leads one to wonder, given the staggeringly enormous death rate, how many great writers, thinkers, scholars and potential world-changers – or ancestors of world-changers – we perhaps lost to the Black Death, and how different our history might look if this terrifying disease had not taken millions of people. The four young daughters of Thomas and Martha Deen in Kent, for example, or the four young daughters of Joan Wynecote née Kerdyf in Worcestershire, or the four older siblings of Agnes Stokwell in London. What might these children have achieved if the pestilence had not stolen their lives so early? Who might their great-great-great-grandchildren have been? Might some of John Wycliffe's contemporaries at the universities of Oxford and Cambridge, who unlike him did succumb to the pestilence, have changed the world with their ideas and their pushing the boundaries of scholarship?

Some of the children and young people who experienced the first pandemic of the Black Death in 1348/49, and whose stories are told here, lived into the 1400s: Julian of Norwich (*c.* 1342–*c.* 1416), Roger Hillary (1331–1400),

Stephen Wynslade (*c.* 1331–1404), John Aylesbury (1334–1409), John Pouger (1336–1405), William Horewode (1342–1422), John Lovell (1342–1408), William Hopegras (*c.* 1343–*c.* 1420), Elizabeth Planke (1348–1423), the sisters Maud Friston (1341/42–1416) and Margaret Friston (*c.* 1344–1422), Thomas Walden (1345–1420) and Thomas Elsing (1346/47–1431). Thomas Elsing announced that he had come of age in February 1368, so was born in or not long before February 1347, perhaps in late 1346. He lost his parents Robert and Alianore and his paternal grandfather William Elsing in 1349/50, and was 85 years old or almost when he finally died in November 1431, surely one of the very last people in England – if not the absolute last – who had lived through the first pandemic of the Black Death. Born twenty years into Edward III's fifty-year reign, Thomas died in the reign of Edward's great-great-grandson Henry VI (r. 1422–61). As well as several outbreaks of the pestilence, he lived through momentous events: the prince of Wales's defeat and capture of King John II of France at the battle of Poitiers in 1356 and John's subsequent incarceration in England, the Peasants' Revolt of 1381, Richard II's abdication in 1399, Henry V's victory over the French at the battle of Agincourt in 1415 and the burning of Joan of Arc in May 1431, six months before he died. A manor-house that Thomas owned in Enfield called Elsyng Palace later belonged to Henry VIII, and the house was rebuilt in the 1620s and renamed Forty Hall. It still stands today. Some remains of Elsyng Spital, the hospital founded by Thomas's grandfather William Elsing in 1330, also survive to this day in central London, and provide another tangible connection to this long-lived survivor of the most catastrophic disease in human history.

Abbreviations

CCR: Calendar of Close Rolls
CFR: Calendar of Fine Rolls
CIM: Calendar of Inquisitions Miscellaneous
CIPM: Calendar of Inquisitions Post Mortem
CLB E: Calendar of Letter-Books of the City of London, Letter-Book E (1314–1337)
CLB F: Calendar of Letter-Books of the City of London, Letter-Book F (1337–1352)
CLB G: Letter-Book G (1352–1374)
CLB H: Letter-Book H (1375–1399)
CPL: Calendar of Entries in the Papal Registers Relating to Great Britain and Ireland: Papal Letters
CPMR: Calendar of Plea and Memoranda Rolls
CPR: Calendar of Patent Rolls
LAN: London Assize of Nuisance 1301–1431
ODNB: Oxford Dictionary of National Biography
TNA: The National Archives
Wills: Calendar of Wills Proved and Enrolled in the Court of Husting, London

Notes

Introduction

1. *Calendar of Wills Proved and Enrolled in the Court of Husting, London*, vol. 1, 1258–1358, ed. Reginald R. Sharpe, 640; *Calendar of Letter-Books of the City of London, Letter-Book G* (1337–52), ed. Reginald R. Sharpe, 229. For what became of Agnes, see Chapter 20.
2. *Polychronicon Ranulphi Higden Monachi Cestrensis*, vol. 8, ed. Joseph Rawson Lumby, 346.
3. John Kelly, *The Great Mortality: An Intimate History of the Black Death* (2005), 11–12.
4. As well as the many books and articles on the subject, novels which feature the Black Death include Connie Willis's *Doomsday Book* (1992), where a student from the 2050s travels back in time to Oxfordshire in 1348, and Karen Maitland's *Company of Liars* (2008), which tells the story of a group of disparate travellers fleeing towards the north of England in the summer and autumn of 1348 after the arrival of the plague on the south coast. Though it was marketed as straight historical fiction, the world depicted in *Company of Liars* is a supernatural and fantastical version of England rather than an accurate portrayal of what the country was really like in the fourteenth century. *Doomsday Book*, though half of it takes place in the 2050s, was written in the late 1980s and did not anticipate modern technology, with the curious result that the sections set in a futuristic England which has invented time travel feel like the 1950s rather than the 2050s. The world of 1348 presented in both novels is a clichéd one where people are dirty, primitive, superstitious and cruel, where undersized girls of 12 are married off to men old enough to be their grandfathers, and where 'the contemps' anachronistically burn witches with gusto.

Chapter 1

1. *Polychronicon Ranulphi Higden*, vol. 8, 344–46. Most of the period from the autumn of 1347 until the spring of 1350 was wet. The winter of 1347/48 saw lots of flooding, the rainy summer of 1348 was followed by another very wet winter in 1348/49, and the autumn of 1349 and the spring of 1350 were, yet again, wet. Derek Vincent Stern, *A Hertfordshire Demesne of Westminster Abbey*, 100, 166.
2. *The Black Death*, ed. and trans. Rosemary Horrox, 65–66.
3. C.M. Woolgar, *The Great Household in Late Medieval England*, 100; Stella Mary Newton, *Fashion in the Age of the Black Prince*, 34.
4. *Foedera, Conventiones, Litterae et Cujuscunque Generis Acta Publica*, vol. 3, part 1, 1344–61, ed. Thomas Rymer, 155, 157; *Calendar of Patent Rolls 1348–50*, 40; *Register of Edward, the Black Prince*, vol. 4, ed. M.C.B. Dawes, 68–69.
5. *Calendar of Close Rolls 1346–49*, 549; *Foedera 1344–61*, 171. Philip VI of France was Queen Philippa's maternal uncle.
6. W. Mark Ormrod, *Edward III*, 357, for the population estimate.
7. *CCR 1323–27*, 101, 120, 347.
8. *Oxford Dictionary of National Biography*, online edition at www.oxforddnb.com. Britannica.com points out that Langland had 'a deep knowledge of medieval theology and was

fully committed to all the implications of Christian doctrine' (www.britannica.com/biography/William-Langland, accessed 28 March 2024).

9. *ODNB.*
10. www.encyclopedia.com/religion/encyclopedias-almanacs-transcripts-and-maps/trevisa-John, accessed 28 March 2024.
11. *ODNB.*
12. *ODNB.*
13. Newton, *Fashion in the Age of the Black Prince*, 9.
14. Judith M. Bennett and Shannon McSheffrey, 'Early, Erotic and Alien: Women Dressed as Men in Late Medieval London', *History Workshop Journal*, 77 (2014), 5.
15. *Coroners Rolls of the City of London 1300–1378*, ed. Reginald R. Sharpe, 256,
16. *Calendar of Entries in the Papal Registers Relating to Great Britain and Ireland: Papal Letters*, vol. 3, 1342–62, ed. W.H. Bliss and C. Johnson, 262, 430, 513; *ODNB.*
17. *Calendar of Inquisitions Post Mortem 1347–52*, nos. 44, 128; *CIPM 1361–65*, no. 358.
18. *Calendar of Letter-Books of the City of London, Letter-Book G* (1352–74), ed. Reginald R. Sharpe, 270, 285, 310.
19. *The Parliament Rolls of Medieval England*, ed. Chris Given-Wilson et al.
20. *CPR 1348–50, 76*; *Parliament Rolls of Medieval England.* The names of the four rivers were spelt Thamise, Cyvern, Ouse and Trente.
21. *CCR 1346–49*, 54, 61–62, 509; *Memorials of London and London Life in the 13*th, *14*th *and 15*th *Centuries*, ed. H.T. Riley, 230–31.
22. *Calendar of Inquisitions Miscellaneous 1348–77*, nos. 7, 14; *CPR 1345–48*, 397; *CPR 1348–50*, 197–98.
23. *London Assize of Nuisance, 1301–1431: A Calendar*, ed. Helena M. Chew and William Kellaway, nos. 414, 417.
24. *Calendar of Wills Proved and Enrolled in the Court of Husting, London,* vol. 1, ed. Reginald R. Sharpe, 545, 699; *CLB F*, 152, 186; *Wills*, vol. 2, 52; *CPL 1342–62*, 376; CPR 1367–70, 371.
25. *CPL 1342–62*, 268; *Testamenta Vetusta: Being Illustrations from Wills*, vol. 1, ed. Nicholas Harris Nicolas, vol. 1, 179–80; *CPR 1348–50*, 251. Charles IV's daughter Anne of Bohemia, from his fourth and last marriage to Elżbieta of Pomerania, married Edward III's grandson Richard II in 1382.
26. *CIPM 1347–52*, no. 107. Alice was born on or around Christmas Day 1281: *CIPM 1307–17*, no. 279.
27. *Petitions to the Pope 1342–1419*, 133–34, 151; *CPL 1342–62*, 302, 305.
28. *CIPM 1347–52*, nos. 72, 110; *CIPM 1365–69*, no. 382; *CIPM 1370–73*, nos. 61, 63, 65, 80; *Calendar of Fine Rolls 1347–56*, 51, 69, 86; *Wills*, vol. 1, 492–93, 501–02, 551; *Wills*, vol. 2, 207; *CLB F*, 181.
29. *CPR 1348–50*, 1, 81, 270–71; www.medievalgenealogy.org.uk/inquests/abstracts_113.shtml.
30. *CIPM 1347–52*, no. 193; *CIPM 1352–60*, nos. 91, 261, 591; *CIPM 1361–65*, nos. 29, 129, 386; *CIPM 1365–69*, nos. 179, 261, 264, 267, 376, 387; *CIPM 1370–73*, nos. 70, 202; *CIPM 1384–92*, no. 940; *CIPM 1427–32*, nos. 483–84; *CLB F*, 181; *Memorials of London*, 240–41.

Chapter 2

1. *The Black Death*, ed. Horrox, 62–66.
2. *Chronicon Galfridi le Baker de Swynbroke*, ed. E.M. Thompson (1899), 97, 100. Although the date of Joan's death is usually given as September 1348, W.M. Ormrod's article

'The Royal Nursery: A Household for the Younger Children of Edward III', English Historical Review, 120 (2005), 413, cites a document in The National Archives, E 101/391/17. This says that one John Badby returned to England on 1 July after Joan's death, *post mortem eiusdem dominae primo die Julii.*

3. *Foedera 1344–61*, 171–72; *CCR 1346–49*, 590; Horrox, Black Death, 250; Gummer, *Scourging Angel*, 55.
4. Ormrod, *Edward III*, 306 note 28.
5. George Frederick Beltz, *Memorials of the Order of the Garter*, 53–54.
6. *Wills*, vol. 1, 307; *CFR 1347–56*, 70; *CIPM 1336–46*, no. 337; *CIPM 1347–52*, no. 118. Laurence was the great-nephew and co-heir of Marie de St Pol's husband Aymer de Valence (d. 1324). His widow Agnes married a second husband named John Hakelut, and died in 1368.
7. *CFR 1347–56*, 109.
8. *CIPM 1347–52*, nos. 216 (Margaret), 217 (Philip), 428 (Hugh). Hugh's heir was his nephew Edward Despenser, born 1336, and Philip's was his son Philip, born 1342.
9. *CIPM 1347–52*, nos. 223–24; *CIPM 1352–60*, no. 203; *CIPM 1361–65*, nos. 201–02.
10. *CIPM 1347–52*, no. 415.
11. *CIPM 1317–27*, no. 60; *CIPM 1347–52*, nos. 291, 451; *CIPM 1370–73*, no. 220.
12. *CIPM 1327–36*, no. 395; *CIPM 1347–52*, no. 379; *CIPM 1352–60*, no. 195.

Chapter 3

1. *CIPM 1347–52*, no. 117; *CFR 1272–1307*, 409; *CCR 1307–13*, 93–94.
2. *CIPM 1327–36*, no. 141; *CIPM 1336–46*, nos. 451–52, 489; *CIPM 1347–52*, no. 123; *CIPM 1352–60*, nos. 508, 618–20; *CIPM 1361–65*, nos. 103, 547, 642; *CIPM 1370–73*, nos. 65, 290; *CIPM 1377–84*, nos. 420–26; *CIPM 1418–22*, nos. 323–27; *CCR 1327–30*, 336; *CCR 1343–46*, 105; *CCR 1346–49*, 507, 570; *CCR 1360–64*, 12–13, 87, 503; *CCR 1381–85*, 287–88; *CFR 1337–47*, 321, 328–29, 359, 368, 380; *CFR 1356–68*, 181–82; Randolph Jones, 'Sir Hugh Tyrell and the French Raid on the Isle of Wight, August 1377', available on Academia.edu.
3. Gummer, *Scourging Angel*, 57.
4. *CIPM 1347–52*, nos. 115, 564; *CFR 1347–56*, 71, 259.
5. *CFR 1356–68*, 202; *CIPM 1361–65*, no. 245; *CIPM 1370–73*, no. 67; *CCR 1369–74*, 221.
6. *CIPM 1384–91*, nos. 988–91; *CCR 1389–92*, 240; CIPM 1427–32, nos. 195–98; *CCR 1429–35*, 7–8. John the younger married a woman called Florence and had a daughter and heir Elizabeth, born *c.* 1415.
7. *CIPM 1352–60*, no. 55; *CIPM 1365–69*, no. 259; *CFR 1347–56*, 361.
8. *CIPM 1361–65*, nos. 169, 379; *CFR 1356–68*, 215.
9. *CIPM 1347–52*, no. 185; *CIPM 1352–60*, nos. 273, 280, 339; *CIPM 1361–65*, nos. 169, 452; *CIPM 1370–73*, nos. 152, 167; *CFR 1347–56*, 115, 221, 398; *CCR 1354–60*, 246–47; *CCR 1360–64*, 365–66; *Feet of Fines for the County of Somerset 1347–1399*, ed. Emanuel Green, 128.
10. *CIPM 1347–52*, no. 212.
11. *CIPM 1327–36*, nos. 550, 692; *CIPM 1347–52*, no. 509; *CFR 1319–27*, 58; *CCR 1333–37*, 552–53.
12. *CIPM 1327–36*, no. 524; *CIPM 1336–46*, no. 218; *CFR 1337–47*, 115, 124, 317; *CFR 1347–56*, 263, 352–53; *CPR 1340–43*, 90, 454; *CIPM 1352–60*, nos. 275, 532, 562; *CCR 1354–60*, 141; *CCR 1364–68*, 248; *CIPM 1361–65*, no. 449; *CIPM 1365–69*, no. 23; *CIPM 1405–13*, nos. 444–45, and for Nicholas Walsh's daughters, see Chapter 20.

13. *CIPM 1347–52*, no. 496; *CFR 1347–56*, 211.
14. *CIPM 1347–52*, nos. 244, 665; *CIPM 1365–69*, nos. 91, 143; *CCR 1364–68*, 321. Richard Lovell's heir in 1351 was his 19-year-old granddaughter Muriel, married to Nicholas Seymour; see Chapter 21.
15. *CIPM 1347–52*, nos. 63, 160–65; *CIPM 1352–60*, no. 534; *CIPM 1384–92*, nos. 1084–91; *CIPM 1392–99*, nos. 442–49; *CIPM 1405–13*, no. 999; *CIPM 1432–37*, nos. 184–90; *CFR 1347–56*, 114, 217, 246, 309–10.
16. *CIPM 1327–36*, no. 540; *CIPM 1347–52*, no. 353; Pierre Gaite, 'The Role and Identity of Household Knights in Fourteenth-Century England, c. 1320–c. 1370', Cardiff Univ. PhD thesis (2020), 42–43, 48, 108, 116, 193, 213.
17. *CPR 1334–38*, 194; The National Archives E 135/24/72.
18. *CIPM 1352–60*, nos. 232, 611; *CFR 1347–56*, 113, 205, 211, 361, 373; *CFR 1356–68*, 135, 141; *CCR 1360–64*, 73, 75, 133–34; *CCR 1369–74*, 119–20; *CIPM 1399–1405*, no. 1138; *CIPM 1422–27*, nos. 125–26.
19. *CIPM 1272–91*, no. 590; *CIPM 1291–1300*, no. 31; *CIPM 1300–07*, no. 44; *CIPM 1307–17*, no. 421; *CIPM 1317–27*, nos. 62, 310; *CIPM 1327–36*, no. 540; Cornwall Record Office, AR/37/5; *CFR 1307–19*, 36; *CPR 1313–17*, 56; *CPR 1321–24*, 181; *CCR 1323–27*, 223.
20. *CIPM 1347–52*, no. 663; *CIPM 1352–60*, no. 384; *CIPM 1361–65*, no. 389.
21. *CIPM 1327–36*, no. 76; *CIPM 1336–46*, no. 483; *CIPM 1347–52*, no. 326; *CIPM 1361–65*, no. 571; *CIPM 1370–73*, no. 153; *CIPM 1392–99*, no. 284; *CCR 1343–46*, 42; *CFR 1347–56*, 112, 119, 294; *CCR 1364–68*, 157.
22. *CIPM 1307–17*, no. 263; *CIPM 1347–52*, nos. 44, 128, 464, 664; *CIPM 1361–65*, no. 358; *CCR 1360–64*, 468.
23. *CIPM 1361–65*, nos. 192, 615; *CIPM 1377–84*, nos. 592–96; *ODNB*.
24. *CIPM 1307–27*, no. 514; *CIPM 1336–46*, nos. 275, 364–65; *CIPM 1347–52*, no. 595; *CIPM 1374–77*, nos. 79, 166; *CIPM 1384–92*, nos. 214–15; *CCR 1381–85*, 442.
25. *CIPM 1347–52*, no. 310; *CIPM 1352–60*, nos. 173, 244.
26. *CIPM 1347–52*, no. 130.

Chapter 4

1. *CIPM 1347–52*, no. 648.
2. Constance Bullock-Davies, *Menestrellorum Multitudo: Minstrels at a Royal Feast*, 186.
3. *CIPM 1291–1300*, no. 404; *CPR 1292–1301*, 417.
4. *CIPM 1347–52*, no. 190; *CIPM 1361–65*, no. 592; *CFR 1347–56*, 209.
5. *CIPM 1347–52*, nos. 149–50; *CFR 1347–56*, 111, 115, 142; *CCR 1349–54*, 10.
6. *CIPM 1300–07*, nos. 116, 133; CIPM 1327–36, no. 410; *CIPM 1347–52*, no. 273; *CIPM 1361–65*, no. 283; *CIPM 1399–1405*, no. 680; *CFR 1327–37*, 304, 309; *CCR 1360–64*, 320–21, 326.
7. *CIPM 1336–46*, no. 678; *CIPM 1347–52*, no. 493; *CIPM 1352–60*, nos. 423, 512; *CFR 1347–56*, 33, 111, 125, 159, 209–10; *CCR 1369–74*, 89; *Abstracts of Feet of Fines*, CP 25/1/288/47, no. 626.
8. *CIPM 1347–52*, no. 327; *CCR 1364–68*, 139, 384.
9. *CIPM 1347–52*, no. 341; *CFR 1347–56*, 129, 215.
10. *CIPM 1327–36*, no. 26; *CIPM 1347–52*, nos. 103, 218, 530; *CIPM 1361–65*, no. 130; *CIPM 1377–84*, nos. 153–57, 866, 868–81; *CIPM 1422–27*, nos. 284–90; *CCR 1377–81*, 168; *CCR 1381–85*, 479–80; *Abstracts of Inquisitiones Post Mortem for Gloucestershire*, vol. 6, 1359–1413, ed. Ethel Stokes, 195–96, 201–02.

11. *CIPM 1307–27*, nos. 98, 538; *CFR 1272–1307*, 295, 297; *CFR 1307–19*, 35.
12. *CIPM 1307–27*, no. 585; *CFR 1307–19*, 35, 38, 253, 259, 276; *CCR 1313–18*, 245.
13. *CIPM 1327–36*, no. 339.
14. *CCR 1323–27*, 419, 423, 532; *CPR 1324–27*, 206; TNA E 40/398; *CPR 1327–30*, 439.
15. *CFR 1327–37*, 246, 272; *CCR 1330–33*, 256; *CIPM 1327–36*, no. 339.
16. *CPR 1343–45*, 19; *CCR 1349–54*, 52–53.
17. *CPR 1348–50*, 275, 317.
18. *CIPM 1347–52*, nos. 251–52, 440; *CCR 1349–54*, 52–53, 125; *CFR 1347–56*, 113, 161, 168, 210, 248; *CIPM 1365–69*, no. 366; *CIPM 1392–99*, nos. 473, 747; *CCR 1392–96*, 47, 334–35.

Chapter 5

1. *CIPM 1361–65*, no. 5; *CIPM 1365–69*, no. 390; *CCR 1369–74*, 122–23.
2. *CIPM 1365–69*, no. 383; *CIPM 1374–77*, no. 301; *CIPM 1384–92*, no. 947.
3. *CIPM 1347–52*, nos. 457–58; *CCR 1349–54*, 184–85, 447; *CCR 1354–60*, 655.
4. *CIPM 1347–52*, no. 324; *CCR 1349–54*, 124.
5. *CIPM 1347–52*, no. 121.
6. www.gatehouse-gazetteer.info/English%20sites/4291.html; www.ecastles.co.uk/westonsubedge.html.
7. *CIPM 1365–69*, no. 21, 22, 186.
8. *CIPM 1365–69*, no. 94.
9. *CIPM 1352–60*, no. 425; *CIPM 1365–69*, nos. 11, 187.
10. *CIPM 1365–69*, nos. 25, 146, 188.
11. *CCR 1374–77*, 173; *CIPM 1374–77*, no. 301.
12. *CIPM 1347–52*, nos. 23, 445, 679; *CIPM 1365–69*, nos. 439, 456.
13. *CIPM 1347–52*, no. 516.
14. *CIPM 1327–36*, no. 658; *CIPM 1336–46*, no. 461; *CIPM 1347–52*, no. 175; *CIPM 1352–60*, no. 332; *CIPM 1365–69*, nos. 12, 456; *CIPM 1374–77*, no. 301.
15. *CIPM 1347–52*, nos. 152, 262; *CIPM 1352–60*, no. 205; *CIPM 1361–65*, no. 391; *CCR 1349–54*, 158.
16. *CIPM 1307–17*, nos. 45, 139, 458; *CIPM 1352–60*, no. 437; *CCR 1323–27*, 405, 407. Ellen and Maud's youngest sister Elizabeth Zouche, born *c.* 1294, became a nun at Brewode Priory. Ellen Cherleton née Zouche had two children from her first marriage: Thomas Seymour (1304–58) and Beatrice, who had a son called John Worth in the late 1330s and died before her brother.
17. *CIPM 1347–52*, no. 459; *CIPM 1352–60*, nos. 320, 503, 606; *CIPM 1361–65*, no. 131; *CIPM 1374–77*, nos. 57, 211; CIPM 1377–84, no. 329; CIPM 1392–99, no. 304; CIPM 1405–13, no. 611; CPR 1358–61, 193; *CPR 1361–64*, 68; *CCR 1364–68*, 83; *CFR 1377–83*, 259; Feet of Fines, CP 25/1/288/47, no. 630; *CIM 1348–77*, nos. 840, 873.
18. *CIPM 1347–52*, nos. 199–200.
19. *CIPM 1300–07*, no. 107; *CIPM 1317–27*, no. 269; *CIPM 1352–60*, no. 372; *CIPM 1361–65*, no. 189; *CIPM 1377–84*, nos. 161–62, 570, 830–31; *CIPM 1392–99*, nos. 667–68; *CIPM 1427–32*, no. 321; *CIPM 1432–37*, nos. 191–92, 401; *CIPM 1442–47*, no. 164; *CPR 1301–07*, 160; *CFR 1319–27*, 29, 36–37; *CFR 1347–56*, 122; *CFR 1377–83*, 126, 128, 153–54, 303, 375; *CFR 1391–99*, 179, 186; *CCR 1318–23*, 22, 250; *CCR 1339–41*, 656; *CCR 1349–54*, 108; *CCR 1369–74*, 136.

Chapter 6

1. *CIPM 1336–46,* nos. 27, 467–68; *CIPM 1347–52*, no. 397.
2. *CPR 1317–21*, 278; *CCR 1318–23*, 150–51; TNA SC 8/259/12929; *CIPM 1307–17*, no. 212.
3. *CIPM 1352–60*, nos. 505, 593; *CIPM 1377–84*, nos. 241–42. Christina's heir was her cousin Nicholas Berenger, son of her father's younger brother,
4. *CIPM 1347–52*, nos. 83, 356–57; *CIPM 1361–65*, no. 540; *CFR 1347–56*, 69, 81–82, 121, 169; *CCR 1360–64*, 464.
5. *Abstracts of Feet of Fines for Wiltshire for the Reign of Edward III*, ed. C.R. Elrington, no. 116.
6. *CIPM 1347–52*, nos. 409–10; *CFR 1347–56*, 117; *CCR 1349–54*, 112.
7. *CIPM 1384–92*, no. 437; *CIPM 1405–13*, no. 786, which states that William was 68 in 1409.
8. *A History of the County of Wiltshire*, vol. 4, available on British History Online, accessed 19 November 2023.
9. TNA BCM/B/4/6/7, 8, 10 and 11 [Berkeley Castle Muniments]; TNA E 40/14748; Wiltshire and Swindon History Centre, 9/14/10, 9/12/5, 9/6/66, 9/6/68, 9/21/4; *CPR 1402–05*, 511; *CIPM 1392–99*, no. 80; *CIPM 1399–1405*, no. 837; *CIPM 1405–13*, nos. 621, 987; *CIPM 1413–18*, no. 807.
10. *CIPM 1413–18*, no. 807; *CCR 1422–29*, 75; hungerfordvirtualmuseum.co.uk, article on Hopgrass Farm, accessed 19 November 2023.
11. *CIPM 1307–17*, no. 317; *CIPM 1317–27*, no. 527; *CFR 1307–19*, 104; *CCR 1323–27*, 215; *CCR 1327–30*, 552; *CPR 1330–34*, 310.
12. *CIPM 1347–52*, no. 242; *CFR 1347–56*, 117, 266; *CCR 1349–54*, 115.
13. *CIPM 1347–52*, no. 311; *CIPM 1352–60*, no. 529; *CIPM 1370–73*, nos. 217, 219; *CCR 1354–60*, 588; *CFR 1356–68*, 198, 202.
14. *CIPM 1347–52*, nos. 222–23; *CCR 1349–54*, 153–55.
15. *CIPM 1347–52*, no. 202.
16. *CIPM 1327–36*, no. 142; *CIPM 1347–52*, no. 112; *CIPM 1352–60*, nos. 317, 370; *CFR 1347–56*, 72, 314; *CFR 1356–68*, 16, 54; *CCR 1333–37*, 372; *CCR 1349–54*, 184, 317, 599; *CCR 1354–60*, 340, 347, 371.
17. *CIPM 1347–52*, nos. 187, 528, 599; *CCR 1349–54*, 49; Feet of Fines, CP 25/1/20/98, no. 11.
18. *CIPM 1347–52*, no. 570; *CIPM 1365–69*, no. 88; *CIPM 1384–92*, nos. 1093–97; *CCR 1389–92*, 453.
19. *CIPM 1370–73*, nos. 38, 71.
20. *CIM 1348–77*, no. 258.
21. *CIPM 1336–46*, no. 122; *CIPM 1347–52*, nos. 207, 390; *CIPM 1352–60*, no. 357; *CIPM 1361–65,* nos. 110, 164, 469; *CCR 1341–43*, 191.

Chapter 7

1. *CIPM 1347–52*, nos. 448–49, 579; *CCR 1346–49*, 25, 64, 175; *CCR 1349–54*, 195; *CFR 1347–56*, 160, 211; *CPR 1348–50, 565*.
2. TNA SC 8/42/2054, SC 8/50/2492.
3. *CIPM 1347–52*, nos. 207–08; *CFR 1347–56*, 115, 139–41, 143; *CCR 1327–30*, 461; *CPR 1327–30*, 192, 565; *CIPM 1418–22*, no. 903.
4. *CIPM 1307–27*, nos. 273, 599; *CIPM 1347–52*, nos. 104, 245, 487.
5. *CIPM 1347–52*, nos. 428, 554, 670; *CFR 1347–56*, 281, 292.

6. *CIPM 1347–52*, no. 597; *CCR 1349–54*, 310; *CCR 1381–85*, 588–89.
7. *CIPM 1347–52*, nos. 287, 370, 394, 497; *CIM 1348–77*, no. 78. For William and Laurence's relationship, see my http://edwardthesecond.blogspot.com/2021/02/laurence-hastings-earl-of-pembroke-d.html.
8. *CIPM 1347–52*, nos. 28, 100; *CIPM 1352–60*, nos. 635–36; *CIPM 1370–73*, no. 195; *Wills*, vol. 1, 499–500, 539; *Wills*, vol. 2, 168; *CFR 1347–56*, 50; *CFR 1356–68*, 133, 147–48, 236, 253; *CLB G*, 38.
9. *CFR 1356–68*, 236, 253; *CCR 1360–64*, 91, 288, 329–30, 481, 534; *Wills*, vol. 2, 120–21; *CIPM 1361–65*, no. 279; *CIPM 1370–73*, no. 195; *LAN*, no. 574; TNA E 326/4290.
10. *Wills*, vol. 1, 499–500; *CCR 1360–64*, 288; *CIPM 1361–65*, nos. 41, 279.
11. *CLB B*, 45; *CLB D*, 141; *CLB E*, 46, 196, 232; *A Descriptive Catalogue of Ancient Deeds*, ed. H.C. Maxwell Lyte, vol. 2, no. B.2885.
12. *CIPM 1327–26*, no. 519; *CIPM 1347–52*, no. 402; *CIPM 1352–60*, no. 118; *CFR 1347–56*, 117.
13. *CFR 1347–56*, 145–46; *CIPM 1347–52*, no. 402; *CCR 1349–54*, 557; *CIPM 1370–73*, no. 195.
14. *CIPM 1399–1405*, nos. 576–77; *CIPM 1405–13*, no. 517; *CIPM 1413–18*, nos. 143–45.
15. *CIPM 1347–52*, no. 184; *CIPM 1365–69*, no. 256; *CIPM 1413–18*, no. 117; *CFR 1347–56*, 158, 200; *CCR 1349–54*, 445–56; *CCR 1364–68*, 493; *CCR 1369–74*, 546.

Chapter 8

1. *Black Death*, ed. Horrox, 65.
2. *Petitions to the Pope*, 234; *CPL 1342–62*, 395–96, 468, 488. In 1354, Walter Manny married Edward III's cousin Margaret of Norfolk, dowager Lady Segrave, and their daughter and heir, Anne Manny, married John Hastings, earl of Pembroke (b. 1347).
3. Barbara E. Megson, 'Mortality Among London Citizens in the Black Death', *Medieval Prosopography*, 19 (1998), 125–33, using *CLB F*, 143; Barney Sloane, *The Black Death in London*, 110.
4. *Memorials of London*, 219, 240.
5. Vincent B. Redstone and Lilian J. Redstone, 'The Heyrons of London: A Study in the Social Origins of Geoffrey Chaucer', *Speculum*, 12 (1937), 185.
6. *CLB E*, 218–19, 226, 237, 239–40; TNA SC 8/169/8432.
7. *Wills*, vol. 1, 360, 600; *Life Records of Chaucer*, nos. 29, 31, 41.
8. *Wills*, vol. 1, 341, 544, 576, 590, 603.
9. *Life Records of Chaucer*, no. 25; *Wills*, vol. 1, 603, 649–51..
10. *CIPM 1365–69*, no. 266.
11. *CPR 1313–17*, 382.
12. *Wills*, 609–10; *CIPM 1347–52*, no. 183; *CIPM 1365–69*, no. 162; *CIPM 1374–77*, no. 172; *CCR 1349–54*, 249; *CCR 1360–64*, 318–19, 394–6; *CCR 1374–77*, 107–08, 201–02, 411; *CLB F*, 158.
13. *Wills*, vol. 1, 361, 515–16.
14. Wills, vol. 1, 612, 615; *Wills*, vol. 2, 167–68; *CIPM 1365–69*, no. 100; *CCR 1374–77*, 219, 280.
15. *CLB D*, 125; *CLB F*, 191–92; *Wills*, 568–69.
16. *Wills*, vol. 1, 531–32, 573, 576, 582, 597.
17. *Wills*, vol. 1, 467–68, 625–26; *Wills*, vol. 2, 77, 174, 388–89; *Memorials of London*, 248–49, 310; *CLB F*, 203; *CLB G*, 141.
18. *Wills*, vol. 1, 312, 485.

19. *Wills*, vol. 1, 611, 614.
20. *CCR 1354–60*, 410; *CIPM 1352–60*, no. 118; *CLB E*, 102.
21. *Wills*, vol. 1, 412, 434, 474, 600, 602.
22. *Calendar of the Plea and Memoranda Rolls*, vol. 1, 201, 209; *Wills*, vol. 1, 543, 563; *CLB F*, 38, 96–97, 211; *CLB G*, 79.
23. *Wills*, vol. 1, 534; *LAN*, no. 361.

Chapter 9

1. *Wills*, vol. 1, 552; *CPR 1338–40*, 105.
2. *Wills*, vol. 1, 509, 559.
3. *Wills*, vol. 1, 551, 563; *Wills*, vol. 2, 295; *CLB E*, 210.
4. *Wills*, vol. 1, 596; *Wills*, vol. 2, 116, 183; *CLB F*, 194, 216; *CLB G*, 219.
5. *Wills*, vol. 1, 411, 534; *CLB F*, 177, 200, 221; *CLB G*, 26, 1546.
6. *Wills*, vol. 1, 517.
7. *Wills*, vol. 1, 408, 425, 555, 622.
8. *Wills*, vol. 1, 417, 494, 542.
9. C LB E, 130; *Wills*, vol. 1, 359, 361, 496, 572, 621–22, 694; *Memorials of London*, 118; *CCR 1349–54*, 353.
10. *CPMR*, vol. 1, 242; *Wills*, vol. 1, 537–38; *CLB F*, 241–42.
11. *Wills*, vol. 1, 532, 560, 622.
12. *Wills*, vol. 1, 291, 515, 540, 580.
13. *Wills*, vol. 1, 558, 560–61, 576; *CLB G*, 8, 145–46; D.J. Keene and Vanessa Harding, *Historical Gazetteer of London Before the Great Fire Cheapside; Parishes of All Hallows Honey Lane, St Martin Pomary, St Mary Le Bow, St Mary Colechurch and St Pancras Soper Lane* (1987), 605–06.
14. *CLB E*, 81–82, 88–89, 170; *Wills*, vol. 1, 223, 273; *Wills*, vol. 2, 320.
15. *Wills*, vol. 1, 593; *CCR 1346–49*, 271; *CCR 1399–1402*, 290; *CPMR*, vol. 1, 275–76; *CPMR*, vol. 2, 51.
16. *CIPM 1361–65*, no. 268; *Wills*, vol. 1, 581, 594, 607–08, 657–59; *CPR 1361–64*, 238–39.
17. *Wills*, vol. 1, 608; *CLB G*, 125; CPMR, vol. 1, 269; *A Descriptive Catalogue of Ancient Deeds*, vol. 2, no. A2359.
18. *Wills*, vol. 1, 596.
19. *Wills*, vol. 1, 388, 618–19.
20. Jordan was the nephew of Alice Brandon, who made her will on 20 March 1349 and died before 9 November; Alice was William Elsing's sister. *Wills*, vol. 1, 362, 376, 548, 562, 612–13, 637, 684; *Wills*, vol. 2, 456; *CPR 1330–34*, 49, 173; *CPR 1340–43*, 415–16; CLB G, 18, 44, 238; John Watney, *Some Account of the Hospital of St Thomas of Acon, in the Cheap, London, and of the Plate of the Mercers' Company* (1892), 247.
21. *CLB F*, 202–03.
22. *Wills*, vol. 1, 572; vol. 2, 23; *CIPM 1336–46*, no. 576; *CPR 1334–38*, 229; *CCR 1339–41*, 21; *CPR 1343–46*, 613; *CCR 1346–49*, 353; *CCR 1364–68*, 398.
23. *Wills*, vol. 1, 599–600; *Wills*, vol. 2, 420–21 (Joan Coterel's son John Body the younger died in 1420); *CPMR*, vol. 3, 138–39; *CCR 1369–74*, 427. John Coterel and his brothers Thomas and Richard were the sons of Richard Coterel, a cordwainer (maker of leather shoes), who died in 1333, and his wife Edith: *Wills*, vol. 1, 389.

Chapter 10

1. *CIPM 1291–1300*, no. 138; *CIPM 1307–17*, no. 59; *CIPM 1336–46*, no. 138; *CIPM 1347–52*, nos. 141–42, 413–14, 431, 643; CIPM 1361–65, no. 549; *CCR 1307–13*, 4; *CFR 1347–56*, 112, 114, 123, 153, 212, 436; *CCR 1349–54*, 142; *CCR 1360–64*, 506; *CPR 1381–85*, 442.
2. *CPR 1358–61*, 172, 445; *CIPM 1361–65*, nos. 235, 549; *CIPM 1365–69*, no. 127; *CIPM 1377–84*, nos. 467–69, 951; *CIPM 1384–92*, no. 79; *An Abstract for the Feet of Fines for the County of Sussex*, vol. 3, ed. L.F. Salzmann (1916), no. 1836. In January 1362 shortly after Edward de Bohun died, his father John de Bohun, now 60 years old, became a father again when his second wife Cecily Filliol – John Lisle III's godmother and step-grandmother – gave birth to a son also named John. The boy was almost four decades younger than his half-sister Joan Lisle.
3. *CIPM 1365–69*, no. 373; *CCR 1369–74*, 48.
4. Feet of Fines CP 25/1/290/60, no. 58; *CCR 1399–1402*, 368. Edmund Dudley (d. 1510), father of John Dudley, duke of Northumberland, and grandfather of Robert Dudley, was the son of Elizabeth Bramshott (d. 1498), Elizabeth Lisle's great-granddaughter: *CIPM 1506–09*, no. 489.
5. *CIPM 1347–52*, nos. 388–89, 655; *CCR 1349–54*, 119–20, 126, 294; *CFR 1347–56*, 156, 286; *CFR 1356–68*, 189–90, 195; *CIPM 1361–65*, no. 226.
6. *CIPM 1336–46*, no. 554; *CIPM 1352–60*, no. 54; *CFR 1347–56*, 396.
7. *CPL 1342–62*, 262.
8. *CPR 1334–38*, 576.
9. *CIPM 1300–07*, no. 422; *CCR 1318–23*, 287, 390.
10. *CPR 1340–43*, 547; *CCR 1346–49*, 173.
11. *CIPM 1347–52*, no. 506; *CIPM 1365–69*, no. 183; *CFR 1347–56*, 111, 210, 247; *CCR 1364–68*, 361.
12. *CIPM 1336–46*, no. 522; *CIPM 1347–52*, nos. 278, 320; *CFR 1347–56*, 153; *CCR 1349–54*, 115; *Inquisitions and Assessments Relating to Feudal Aids 1284–1431*, vol. 2, 337, 339.
13. *CIPM 1327–36*, no. 112; *CIPM 1347–52*, 312; *CCR 1349–54*, 176; *CFR 1347–52*, no. 161; *Feet of Fines*, CP 25/1/289/52, no. 16.
14. *CIPM 1347–52*, no. 220–21, 451, 581, 680; *CFR 1347–56*, 173, 259–60, 264; *CCR 1349–54*, 23; *CCR 1354–60*, 467–68.
15. *CIPM 1370–73*, no. 69.
16. *CIPM 1347–52*, no. 131.

Chapter 11

1. *CIPM 1336–46*, no. 666; *CIPM 1347–52*, nos. 124, 215; *CPR 1345–48*, 203, 223; *CCR 1346–49*, 481; *CFR 1337–47*, 479, 494–95; CFR 1347–56, 117, 221.
2. *CIPM 1272–91*, no. 686.
3. *CIPM 1347–52*, no. 629; *CIPM 1352–60*, no. 208; *CCR 1354–60*, 153.
4. *CIPM 1347–52*, no. 272; *CIPM 1352–60*, no. 410; *CFR 1347–56*, 119.
5. *CIPM 1317–27*, no. 148; *CIPM 1336–46*, no. 74; *CFR 1307–19*, 375, 399.
6. *LAN*, nos. 263, 288.
7. *Coroners Rolls*, 119–20; *CPR 1324–27*, 200; *CCR 1337–39*, 293–94.
8. TNA SC 8/203/10108 and 10109; *CFR 1319–27*, 64; *CCR 1318–23*, 313–14, 403–04; *CLB E*, 121.
9. *CIPM 1336–46*, nos. 94, 189; *CFR 1337–47*, 20, 63; *CCR 1337–39*, 290, 293–94, 319–20, 351–52, 405–06; *CPR 1340–43*, 5.

10. *Wills*, vol. 1, 606; *CIPM 1347–52*, no. 272.
11. *CIPM 1347–52*, no. 176.
12. *CIPM 1347–52*, no. 215.
13. *CIPM 1352–60*, no. 196; *CCR 1354–60*, 123.
14. *CIPM 1347–52*, no. 282.
15. *CIPM 1272–91*, no. 11; *CIPM 1317–27*, no. 573; *CIPM 1336–46*, no. 192; *CIPM 1347–52*, nos. 282–83, 574; *CIPM 1361–65*, no. 200; *CPR 1327–30*, 15, 310; *CPR 1330–34*, 103–04, 314; *CFR 1347–56*, 124, 240, 263, 267; *CCR 1349–54*, 286; *CCR 1360–64*, 66–68, 447.
16. *CIPM 1347–52*, nos. 179–80; *CIPM 1352–60*, no. 284; www.british-history.ac.uk/rchme/northants/vol1/pp8-11, accessed 27 December 2023.
17. *CIPM 1347–52*, no. 321; *CIPM 1361–65*, no. 387; *CFR 1347–56*, 188, 240; *CCR 1360–64*, 374.
18. *CIPM 1352–60*, no. 398; *CFR 1347–56*, 211; *CCR 1349–54*, 133, 184; *CCR 1354–60*, 378.
19. *CIPM 1347–52*, nos. 301, 563; *CIPM 1352–60*, no. 553; *CFR 1347–56*, 162–63, 224, 295–96, 298, 381; *CCR 1360–64*, 2–3.
20. *CIPM 1300–07*, no. 91; *CIPM 1317–27*, nos. 391, 410; *CIPM 1336–46*, no. 687; *CFR 1272–1307*, 461–62; *CFR 1347–56*, 157; East Sussex and Brighton and Hove Record Office GLY/1332.
21. *CIPM 1336–46*, no. 337; *CIPM 1365–69*, no. 18.
22. *CIPM 1327–36*, no. 652; *CIPM 1336–46*, no. 89; *CIPM 1347–52*, no. 178; *CIPM 1352–60*, nos.166, 367; *CIPM 1365–69*, nos. 18, 112; *CIPM 1413–18*, nos. 49, 260–62; *CIPM 1418–22*, nos. 495–97; CIPM 1422–27, nos. 692–93; *CCR 1318–23*, 427; *CFR 1319–27*, 187–88, 197, 206–07; *CFR 1347–56*, 117, 123, 157, 183, 250; *CCR 1364–68*, 347–48; *CCR 1374–77*, 35.

Chapter 12

1. *CIPM 1370–73*, no. 65; *CPR 1405–08*, 442; *Testamenta Vetusta*, 171; *CIPM 1413–18*, 32.
2. *CIPM 1336–46*, no. 317; *CIPM 1347–52*, nos. 173, 615; *CIPM 1352–60*, nos. 77, 132, 489; *CIPM 1374–77*, no. 292; *CCR 1349–54*, 118, 123, 169–70, 299–300, 546–47; *CCR 1360–64*, 228–29, 549–50, 553.
3. *CCR 1349–54*, 145. The description of the manor-house is in *CIPM 1418–22*, no. 150.
4. *CIPM 1347–52*, no. 429; *CIPM 1352–60*, no. 262; *CIPM 1405–13*, nos. 683–89; *CCR 1318–23*, 435, 450; *CCR 1330–33*, 428; *CPR 1334–38*, 109; *CFR 1347–56*, 179; *CCR 1381–85*, 250, 283; *CIPM 1418–22*, nos. 93–104, 150, 889–94; *CIPM 1422–27*, nos. 2, 267–68; www.historyofparliamentonline.org/volume/1386-1421/member/aylesbury-sir-john-1334-1409.
5. *CIPM 1327–36*, no. 623; *CIPM 1347–52*, no. 294; *CIPM 1361–65*, nos. 108–09, 196, 378. Warin and Thomas are not specifically stated to have been twins, but Warin, named as their elder brother John's heir, was said to have turned 19 around 10 August 1360 and died before January 1362 when he was still under 21. Thomas's proof of age taken in November 1362 states that he was born on 14 September 1341.
6. *The Complete Peerage*, vol. 7, 455–56; *CIPM 1399–1405*, nos. 435 39, 609–13; *CIPM 1405–13*, 807–09.
7. *CIPM 1336–46*, nos. 407–08; *CIPM 1347–52*, no. 605.
8. *CIPM 1347–52*, nos. 19, 461, 555; *CIPM 1361–65*, no. 69; *CFR 1347–56*, 51, 64, 294.
9. *CIPM 1347–52*, no. 621.
10. *Wills*, vol. 1, 608.

11. *CIPM 1347–52*, nos. 283, 447; *CIPM 1361–65*, no. 200; *CCR 1330–33*, 302.
12. *CIPM 1347–52*, no. 230; *CIPM 1361–65*, no. 429; *CCR 1360–64*, 353–54, 510–11; Nicholas Hamilton Bennett, 'The Beneficed Clergy in the Diocese of Lincoln during the Episcopate of Henry Burghersh, 1320–1340', Univ. of York DPhil thesis (1989), vol. 2, Appendix: A Calendar of the Institution Register, no. 2120.
13. *CIPM 1347–52*, no. 641.
14. *CIPM 1347–52*, no. 378; *CIPM 1352–60*, no. 27; *CIPM 1365–69*, no. 348; *CFR 1347–56*, 185.
15. www.bbc.co.uk/history/british/middle_ages/black_01.shtml, accessed 25 January 2024.
16. *Wills*, vol. 1, 463, 514, 519; CLF, 175.
17. *Wills*, vol. 1, 463, 514, 519, 535, 593–94.
18. *CIPM 1347–52*, no. 363.
19. *CIPM 1352–60*, no. 127.

Chapter 13

1. *CIPM 1300–07*, no. 371; *CIPM 1327–36*, no. 709; *CIPM 1336–46*, no. 672; *CCR 1333–37*, 404–05; *CFR 1327–37*, 441, 448–49. William the elder's parents were James Planke and Maud, heiress of Haversham in Buckinghamshire. His elder brother John, born in 1301 and named as their father's heir in 1306, must have died young. William the younger's mother was perhaps a member of the Poyntz family, who held Curry Mallet, his birthplace in 1325.
2. *CIPM 1352–60*, no. 124.
3. *CIPM 1347–52*, nos. 31, 281; *CIPM 1352–60*, nos. 281, 328, 335; *CIPM 1361–65*, no. 126; *CPR 1334–38*, 222; *CCR 1346–49*, 132, 290, 335; *CFR 1347–56*, 27, 55; *CCR 1354–60*, 264–65; *CCR 1360–64*, 233. Elizabeth Planke's proof of age says she was born on 1 January 1346, but several inquisitions make it apparent that her mother was pregnant with her when her father died on 5 September 1347 and that she was born after 6 November 1347.
4. *Testamenta Vetusta*, 61. The church was later dedicated to St Matthew.
5. *CIPM 1377–84*, nos. 420–26; *CIPM 1392–99*, nos. 586, 1122–26; *CIPM 1399–1405*, no. 772.
6. *CIPM 1418–22*, nos. 795–96; *CIPM 1422–27*, nos. 333–45; the heir was William Lucy, descendant of Joan Pabenham née Planke, sister of William Planke who died in 1335.
7. *Records of the Borough of Leicester*, vol. 2, 143, 206–07, 388, 392–93, 401, 405.
8. *CIPM 1336–46*, no. 202; *CIPM 1347–52*, no. 166; *CIPM 1370–73*, no. 70; *CIPM 1384–92*, no. 520; *CFR 1347–56*, 119, 138–39; *CCR 1369–74*, 122, 188.
9. *CIPM 1327–36*, no. 433; *CIPM 1347–52*, no. 153; *CIPM 1361–65*, no. 381; *CIPM 1370–73*, no. 161; *CCR 1349–54*, 115; www.british-history.ac.uk/staffs-hist-collection/vol11/pp176-183.
10. *CIPM 1347–52*, nos. 229, 437; *CFR 1327–37*, 474; *CFR 1337–47*, 85, 139, 168, 200; *CFR 1347–56*, 127, 239; *CPR 1348–50*, 391, 503.
11. *CIPM 1347–52*, no. 428; *CIPM 1361–65*, no. 442; *CIPM 1365–69*, no. 421; *CIPM 1370–73*, no. 128; *CIPM 1374–77*, no. 212.
12. *CIPM 1352–60*, nos. 32, 408; *CCR 1369–74*, 186, 351; *CIPM 1384–92*, no. 558.
13. *CIPM 1347–52*, no. 435; *CFR 1347–56*, 156; *CCR 1349–54*, 251; *CCR 1377–81*, 241.
14. *CIPM 1347–52*, nos. 396, 484; *CIPM 1351–65*, no. 261; *CIPM 1365–69*, nos. 87, 296.
15. *CIPM 1347–52*, nos. 160, 539; *CIPM 1352–60*, no. 119.
16. *CIPM 1347–52*, no. 369.

17. *CIPM 1291–1300*, nos. 136–37, 593; *CIPM 1307–17*, no. 226; CIPM 1336–46, no. 105; *CPR 1292–1301*, 563, 594; *CCR 1307–13*, 516; *CFR 1307–19*, 245; *CCR 1313–18*, 20, 243; *CPR 1334–38*, 47.
18. *CPR 1301–07*, 418, 534; *CPR 1317–21*, 362; *CPR 1321–24*, 3; *CPR 1334–38*, 47–48; *CFR 1337–47*, 57, 66; *CFR 1347–56*, 377–78; *CIPM 1336–46*, no. 105; *CIPM 1352–60*, no. 102; *Staffordshire Historical Collections*, vol. 7, part 1, 113, 136, 162, 167.
19. *CPR 1343–45*, 10; *Staffordshire Historical Collections*, vol. 11, 155.
20. *CIPM 1347–52*, no. 369; *CFR 1347–56*, 153, 181, 185; *CCR 1349–54*, 495; *CIPM 1352–60*, no. 102; *CIPM 1370–73*, no. 271; *CFR 1369–77*, 238.
21. *CIPM 1392–99*, nos. 672–75; *CIPM 1405–13*, nos. 953–54.

Chapter 14

1. *CIPM 1347–52*, nos. 91, 543; *CIPM 1365–69*, nos. 245, 255; CFR 1347–56, 210, 294, 368; *CCR 1369–74*, 2.
2. *CIPM 1384–92*, no. 979.
3. *CIPM 1327–36*, nos. 340, 631; *CIPM 1352–60*, no. 15; *CIPM 1361–65*, no. 214; *CIPM 1365–69*, no. 184. *CFR 1327–37*, 256; *CIPM 1418–22*, no. 547; *CIPM 1437–42*, nos. 364–65; *CIPM 1442–47*, no. 468.
4. *CIPM 1347–52*, nos. 490, 544; *CIPM 1352–60*, no. 124; *CFR 1347–56*, 125, 320; *CCR 1349–54*, 549.
5. *CIPM 1317–27*, no. 210; *CCR 1318–23*, 578; *CFR 1327–37*, 425.
6. *CIPM 1352–60*, no. 526; *CIPM 1361–65*, no. 52; *CFR 1347–56*, 208; CPR 1348–50, 466; *CCR 1349–54*, 131, 215; *CCR 1354–60*, 555.
7. *CIPM 1347–52*, no. 669.
8. *CIPM 1336–46*, no. 521; *CIPM 1347–52*, nos. 135, 423–24; *CIPM 1365–69*, no. 267; *CIPM 1374–77*, nos. 8, 87–88; *CCR 1349–54*, 131, 215; *CFR 1347–56*, 154, 157, 202, 208; *CPR 1348–50*, 283; *CCR 1381–85*, 258.
9. *CIPM 1361–65*, no. 52; *CIPM 1374–77*, no. 104; *CIPM 1377–84*, no. 291; *CCR 1377–81*, 262–63.
10. *CIPM 1374–77*, no. 95; TNA C 143/343/1.
11. *CIPM 1374–77*, nos. 95–96, 104; *CFR 1369–77*, 325–26, 328.
12. *CCR 1374–77*, 172, 456.
13. *CFR 1399–1405*, 270; *CIPM 1422–27*, no. 681. A Richard Baynard was the attorney of Joan Holland, dowager duchess of York, in Middlesex in 1405, though it is impossible to tell whether this is the same man (*CIPM 1399–1405*, no. 1185).
14. *CIPM 1347–52*, no. 617.
15. *CIPM 1347–52*, no. 337; *CCR 1349–54*, 120–21.
16. *CIPM 1327–36*, no. 451; *CIPM 1347–52*, no. 349; *CIPM 1352–60*, nos. 392, 526, 551, 472–73; *CCR 1330–33*, 509; *CCR 1346–49*, 359; *CCR 1349–54*, 193; CCR 1354–60, 376; *CFR 1327–37*, 332; *CFR 1347–56*, 160, 207, 306.
17. *CIPM 1347–52*, no. 125; *CIPM 1352–60*, no. 74; *CFR 1327–37*, 435, 437; *CCR 1333–37*, 398, 560–61; *CCR 1341–43*, 239, 279–80; *CCR 1346–49*, 481; *CPR 1334–38*, 97; *CPR 1338–40*, 107, 116; *Feet of Fines for Essex*, vol. 2, 217. It is possible that Mabel FitzWarin, Queen Philippa's attendant who was granted custody of James Tracy, was his mother, who also bore the name Mabel but whose identity is unclear.
18. *CIPM 1347–52*, no. 518; *CIPM 1352–60*, nos. 104, 363, 400; *CPR 1334–38*, 22, 140; *CFR 1347–56*, 125, 358; *CCR 1339–41*, 227; *CCR 1349–54*, 266–67, 274–75, 472; *CCR 1354–60*, 349; *CCR 1364–68*, 168, 197, 201–03.

19. www.historyofparliamentonline.org/volume/1386-1421/member/marney-sir-robert-1319-1400, accessed 4 October 2023. Marny often appears in the chancery rolls.
20. *CPR 1350–54*, 455; *CPR 1354–58*, 572; *CCR 1364–68*, 201–03; *CIM 1348–77*, no. 142; *CIPM 1352–60*, no. 383.
21. *CLB F*, 199; *CPMR*, vol. 1, 227.
22. *CIPM 1300–07*, no. 174; *CIPM 1327–36*, no. 463; *CIPM 1347–52*, no. 174; *CIPM 1370–73*, no. 329; *CIPM 1392–99*, nos. 66–68; *CIPM 1399–1405*, no. 666; CFR 1347–56, 173, 223; *CCR 1346–49*, 275, 371; *CCR 1399–1402*, 452; TNA C 143/270/14.
23. *CIPM 1347–52*, no. 298; *CIPM 1361–65*, no. 213; *CFR 1347–56*, 121, 254; *CFR 1356–68*, 197, 200, 225; *CCR 1354–60*, 317.
24. *CIPM 1327–36*, no. 542; *CIPM 1336–46*, nos. 237, 376; *CIPM 1352–60*, nos. 127, 468; *CIPM 1365–69*, no. 212; *CIPM 1374–77*, no. 245; *CIPM 1377–84*, no. 308; *CIPM 1432–37*, nos. 62–66.
25. *CIPM 1347–52*, no. 246. There is also a Great Oakley in Northamptonshire.
26. *Wills*, vol. 1, 699–700.
27. *ODNB*.
28. *CIPM 1336–46*, no. 463; *CIPM 1347–52*, nos. 295, 598; John's father, also John Segrave (d. 1343), was the younger brother of Stephen, Lord Segrave (d. 1325).
29. *CIPM 1352–60*, no. 395; *CCR 1354–60*, 358; *CFR 1347–56*, 123, 178.
30. *CIPM 1365–69*, no. 62; *CCR 1364–68*, 224–25, 317–18.
31. *CIPM 1352–60*, no. 395; *CIPM 1365–69*, nos. 308, 327.
32. *CIPM 1336–46*, no. 330; *CIPM 1347–52*, nos. 171–72; *CCR 1313–18*, 89, 237, 283; *CFR 1347–56*, 114, 121.

Chapter 15

1. *CPMR*, vol. 1, 4; *Wills*, vol. 1, 475–76.
2. *CCR 1343–45*, 490; *Wills*, vol. 1, 603, 649–51.
3. *LAN*, nos. 324–26, 328; *CLB F*, 71, 172.
4. *CPMR*, vol. 1, 122–29; *Coroners Rolls*, 266–69; *CPR 1340–43*, 226–27.
5. *Wills*, vol. 1, 603, 649–51; *CLB G*, 129, 136, 145, 158, 228; *CCR 1399–1402*, 419; TNA C 241/183/9.
6. *CIPM 1307–17*, no. 144; *CIPM 1347–52*, nos. 473, 475, 477; *CIPM 1352–60*, nos. 295, 475, 496; *CFR 1307–19*, 41, 43; *CCR 1307–13*, 302; *CCR 1318–23*, 183; *CFR 1356–68*, 15, 23–24; *CCR 1360–64*, 2.
7. *CIPM 1347–52*, no. 479; *CIPM 1361–65*, no. 538; *CCR 1360–64*, 501–02.
8. *CIPM 1347–52*, no. 480; *CIPM 1352–60*, no. 224; *CCR 1354–60*, 132.
9. *CIPM 1327–36*, nos. 510, 549; *CIPM 1347–52*, no. 627; *CIPM 1352–60*, no. 165; *CFR 1347–56*, 159, 372, 396.
10. *CIPM 1352–60*, nos. 352, 463; *CIPM 1361–65*, no. 225.
11. *CIPM 1352–60*, no. 514; *CIPM 1365–69*, no. 86; *CCR 1349–54*, 390; *CCR 1369–74*, 92–93; *CCR 1374–77*, 361.
12. *CIPM 1336–46*, no, 278; *CIPM 1347–52*, nos. 329, 583; *CIPM 1352–60*, nos. 415, 454; *CIPM 1361–65*, no. 431; *CCR 1385–89*, 145.
13. *CIPM 1347–52*, no. 478; *CIPM 1352–60*, no. 479.

Chapter 16

1. *CIPM 1347–52*, nos. 147, 366; *CIPM 1352–60*, no. 423; *CFR 1347–56*, 235; *CPL 1342–62*, 411; *CIM 1348–77*, no. 388.

2. *CIPM 1347–52*, no. 426; *CIPM 1365–69*, no. 176; *CFR 1347–56*, 126.
3. *CIPM 1347–52*, no. 170; *CIPM 1352–60*, no. 159.
4. *CIPM 1336–46*, nos. 529–30, 572, 607; *CIPM 1347–52*, nos. 120, 290–91, 293, 444, 572; *CFR 1347–56*, 125, 177.
5. *CIPM 1327–36*, no. 61; *CIPM 1347–52*, no. 666.
6. *CIPM 1327–36*, no. 691; *CIPM 1336–46*, no. 31; *CIPM 1347–52*, no. 411; *CIPM 1352–60*, nos. 200–01, 245; CCR 1333–37, 609; *CFR 1327–37*, 492; *CFR 1347–56*, 152, 372, 421.
7. *CIPM 1347–52*, no. 134; *CFR 1347–56*, 126; *CCR 1349–54*, 119, 163; *CCR 1381–85*, 361; *CCR 1385–89*, 69–70.
8. *CIPM 1361–65*, no. 545.
9. *CFR 1347–56*, 288, is an order dated 14 November 1351 to take her lands into the king's hands, which was 'vacated because it is testified that Alice is alive'. On 16 November 1351 (*CPR 1350–54*, 181), Alice was called 'late the wife' of Edward Montacute, and was certainly dead by 30 January 1352; *CFR 1347–56*, 345; *CCR 1349–54*, 411–12; *CCR 1354–60*, 222; *CPR 1350–54*, 230; *CPR 1361–64*, 26. See my https://edwardthesecond.blogspot.com/2019/04/the-life-and-tragic-death-of-alice-of.html.
10. *CPR 1350–54*, 181; *CCR 1360–64*, 455.
11. *CIPM 1361–65*, nos. 140–41, 516.
12. *CIPM 1327–36*, no. 419; *CIPM 1347–52*, no. 538; *CIPM 1352–60*, 480; *CIPM 1365–69*, no. 141; *CFR 1327–37*, 365–66; *CFR 1347–56*, 211, 265.
13. *CIPM 1327–36*, nos. 143, 163; *CIPM 1347–52*, no. 243; *CFR 1327–37*, 98, 102, 261, 263: *CCR 1327–30*, 316, 546–47; *CCR 1349–54*, 106.
14. *CIPM 1347–52*, no. 303; *CIPM 1347–52*, nos. 284–85; *CIPM 1352–60*, nos. 13, 573; *CCR 1330–33*, 74; *CCR 1349–54*, 159; *CIPM 1365–69*, no. 15.
15. *CIM 1348–77*, no. 156.
16. *CIPM 1370–73*, no. 136.

Chapter 17

1. *CIPM 1352–60*, no. 555; *Petitions to the Pope*, 529.
2. *CIPM 1347–52*, no. 450; *CIPM 1352–60*, no. 125; *CIPM 1432–37*, no. 273; *CFR 1347–56*, 230; *CCR 1349–54*, 174; *CCR 1354–60*, 2, 151.
3. *ODNB*.
4. *CIPM 1347–52*, nos. 219, 234; Gummer, *Scourging Angel*, 221, 225.
5. *CIPM 1235–72*, no. 633; *CIPM 1272–91*, nos. 553, 637, 819; *CIPM 1291–1300*, no. 540; *CIPM 1317–27*, nos. 198, 591–92; *CIPM 1327–36*, no. 517; *CIPM 1336–46*, nos. 67, 143, 560; *CIPM 1347–52*, nos. 5, 191–92, 195; *CIPM 1352–60*, no. 555; *CIPM 1370–73*, nos. 181–82; *CIPM 1405–13*, nos. 119–22; *CIPM 1413–18*, nos. 552–55; *CIPM 1418–22*, nos. 755–57; *CPR 1327–30*, 109; *CFR 1337–47*, 64, 426; *CFR 1347–56*, 123–24, 164, 173, 175, 233; *CCR 1323–27*, 398, 455; *CCR 1333–37*, 286, 618; *CCR 1354–60*, 348; *CCR 1422–29*, 38, 215.
6. *CIPM 1352–60*, no. 368; *CIPM 1365–69*, no. 382; *CCR 1339–41*, 51–53; *CCR 1341–43*, 210, 258; *CCR 1369–74*, 13; TNA C 143/371/15.
7. *CIPM 1352–60*, nos. 101, 157; *CFR 1347–56*, 372.
8. *CIPM 1317–27*, no. 425; *CIPM 1336–46*, no. 52; *CIPM 1347–52*, no. 226; *CIPM 1352–60*, no. 393; *CCR 1323–27*, 28–38; *CCR 1349–54*, 122, 287, 318, 474; *CFR 1347–56*, 159, 182, 281; *CCR 1402–05*, 122.
9. Gummer, *Scourging Angel*, 222.

10. *CIPM 1347–52*, nos. 93, 143–45, 267, 275, 281, 314, 332, 345, 347, 355, 358–59, 364, 384–85, 442, 452, 455, 618; *CPR 1338–40*, 528; *CFR 1347–56*, 153, 176, 180; *CCR 1349–54*, 175.
11. *CIPM 1336–46*, no. 481; *CIPM 1361–65*, no. 535.
12. *CIPM 1336–46*, no. 500; *CIPM 1347–52*, nos. 325, 382, 453, 602, 616, 620; *CIPM 1365–69*, no. 158; *CCR 1364–68*, 101–02.
13. *CIPM 1317–27*, no. 580; *CIPM 1347–52*, nos. 167–68; *CIPM 1352–60*, no. 651.
14. *CCR 1339–41*, 171–74; *CPR 1338–40*, 66–67.
15. *CIPM 1307–17*, no. 365; *CIPM 1336–46*, nos. 209, 389; *CIPM 1347–52*, nos. 92, 354; *CIPM 1352–60*, nos. 266, 393, 456, 648, 651; *CIPM 1370–73*, no. 326; *CCR 1341–43*, 440; *CCR 1349–54*, 42–43; *CFR 1347–56*, 72, 184.

Chapter 18

1. *CIPM 1336–46*, no. 610; *CIPM 1347–52*, nos. 20, 305; CIPM 1365–69, no. 94; *CCR 1346–49*, 133–34, 232; *CCR 1349–54*, 173; *CFR 1347–56*, 160, 236.
2. *CIPM 1327–36*, nos. 130, 202; *CIPM 1336–46*, nos. 604, 646; *CIPM 1347–52*, no. 313; *CIPM 1361–65*, no. 574; *CIPM 1384–92*, nos. 1001–02; *CFR 1337–47*, 460; *CFR 1347–56*, 124, 160, 282; *CCR 1343–46*, 408, 532; *CCR 1349–54*, 164. The siblings' paternal grandparents were Richard (d. 1345) and Alice (d. 1329).
3. *CIPM 1365–69*, no. 257.
4. *CIPM 1336–46*, no. 642; *CIPM 1361–65*, no. 567; *CIPM 1370–73*, no. 264; *CFR 1356–68*, 285.
5. *CIPM 1347–52*, no. 647; *CIPM 1361–65*, no. 75; *CCR 1360–64*, 224.
6. *CIPM 1317–27*, nos. 130, 404; *CIPM 1327–36*, no. 622; *CIPM 1347–52*, no. 639; *CIPM 1365–69*, no. 147; *CCR 1327–30*, 514.
7. *CPR 1348–50*, 389; *CPR 1350–54*, 19.
8. *CIPM 1365–69*, no. 147; *CFR 1356–68*, 301, 311; *CCR 1364–68*, 340.
9. *CIPM 1352–60*, nos. 36, 44, 459; *CIPM 1361–65*, no. 323; *CIPM 1374–77*, nos. 132, 328; *CIPM 1392–99*, no. 339; *CCR 1360–64*, 5; *CFR 1347–56*, 348; *CFR 1356–68*, 246.
10. *CIPM 1365–69*, no. 90; *CIPM 1405–13*, nos. 386–88; *CIPM 1418–22*, no. 923; *CCR 1377–81*, 72, 163; *CCR 1389–92*, 216, 233, 246; *CPR 1401–05*, 255; *ODNB*.
11. *CIPM 1347–52*, no. 585; *CIPM 1361–65*, no. 382; *CCR 1360–64*, 345.
12. *CIPM 1352–60*, no. 45; *CIPM 1361–65*, no. 133; *CIPM 1377–84*, no. 598; *CFR 1356–68*, 8–9, 73; *CCR 1360–64*, 460; *CCR 1381–85*, 163.
13. *CIPM 1317–27*, no. 387; *CIPM 1336–46*, no. 501; *CIPM 1347–52*, no. 566; *CIPM 1361–65*, nos. 382, 561; *CIPM 1365–69*, no. 59; *CIPM 1413–18*, no. 513; *CIPM 1422–27*, nos. 19, 346; *CCR 1349–54*, 170, 189; *CFR 1356–68*, 278, 288, 335, 344.
14. *CIPM 1361–65*, no. 435; *CCR 1377–81*, 371.
15. *CIPM 1352–60*, no. 405; *CIPM 1365–69*, no. 16; *CCR 1369–74*, 18.
16. *CIPM 1336–46*, no. 609; *CIPM 1347–52*, no. 417; *CFR 1337–47*, 426–27, 437; *CFR 1347–56*, 161, 228; *CCR 1346–49*, 5, 86–88.

Chapter 19

1. *CIPM 1336–46*, nos. 458–59; *CIPM 1347–52*, no. 386; *CIPM 1361–65*, no. 408; *CIPM 1399–1405*, no. 1176; *CCR 1343–46*, 186–87, 195; *CCR 1349–54*, 52, 101; *CCR 1405–09*, 13. Emma Scaleby had a daughter called Alice Wode, who had daughters Margaret Pape and Maud Walker.
2. *CIPM 1347–52*, no. 520; *CIPM 1365–69*, no. 258; *CIPM 1399–1405*, nos. 856, 675; *CCR 1364–68*, 416, 425.

3. *CIPM 1347–52*, no. 521; *CIPM 1361–65*, no. 474; *CCR 1360–64*, 465–66; *CCR 1389–92*, 556.
4. *CIPM 1347–52*, no. 551; *CFR 1347–56*, 239–40; *CCR 1385–89*, 34.
5. *CIPM 1347–52*, no. 524; *CIPM 1352–60*, no. 202; *CCR 1349–54*, 305; *CCR 1364–68*, 413, 418; *CIPM 1432–37*, nos. 402–03, 467–68; *CIPM 1437–42*, nos. 212–15.
6. *CIPM 1347–52*, no. 610; *CIPM 1352–60*, no. 80.
7. *CIPM 1352–60*, no. 290.
8. *CIPM 1365–69*, no. 181.
9. *CIPM 1317–27*, no. 597; *CIPM 1327–36*, no. 615; *CIPM 1365–69*, no. 410; *CIPM 1399–1405*, no. 523; *CCR 1349–54*, 161, 175, 215; *CCR 1374–77*, 398; *CCR 1377–81*, 430, 434–37, 457; *CCR 1385–89*, 142, 275.
10. *CIPM 1327–36*, no. 65; *CIPM 1347–52*, nos. 454, 588; *CIPM 1361–65*, no. 348; *CIPM 1384–92*, nos. 120, 247.
11. *CIPM 1327–36*, nos. 536, 638; *CIPM 1336–46*, nos. 282, 385; *CIPM 1347–52*, no. 211; *CIPM 1361–65*, no. 598; *CIPM 1377–84*, nos. 142–44; *CIPM 1384–92*, nos. 1034–38; *CCR 1307–13*, 138; *CCR 1313–18*, 291; *CPR 1313–17*, 403; *CCR 1333–37*, 238–40, 325; *CCR 1341–43*, 483–84; *CCR 1354–60*, 86, 387, 400, 502, 515, 522; *CCR 1364–68*, 96, 234, 331–32; *CCR 1369–74*, 515, 521; *CCR 1396–99*, 60, 71; *Descriptive Catalogue of Ancient Deeds*, vol. 4, no. A.6866.
12. *CIPM 1361–65*, no. 417; *CIPM 1365–69*, no. 180; *CIPM 1418–22*, nos. 419–20.

Chapter 20

1. *CIPM 1370–73*, no. 68; *CFR 1369–77*, 55, 101; *CCR 1369–74*, 161.
2. *CIPM 1361–65*, no. 328; *CIPM 1370–73*, no. 288; *CCR 1360–64*, 353.
3. *CLB F*, 205, 223–24, 286–87.
4. *CIPM 1370–73*, nos. 179, 303; www.medievalgenealogy.org.uk/inquests/abstracts_113.shtml.
5. *CLB F*, 199, 207, 210, 222; *CPR 1348–50*, 459; *Memorials of London*, 253–58.
6. *CIPM 1370–73*, no. 142.
7. *CIM 1348–77*, no. 26; *CIPM 1361–65*, no. 65; *CIPM 1365–69*, no. 342; *CIPM 1370–73*, no. 139; *CIPM 1374–77*, no. 98; *CIPM 1377–84*, no. 691; *CIPM 1405–13*, no. 541; *CIPM 1422–27*, no. 237; *CIPM 1432–37*, nos. 313–14; *CIPM 1437–42*, nos. 417–19; CFR 1347–56, 211. John's sister Margaret married Robert Fouleshurst and had a son Thomas in about 1370.
8. *CIPM 1370–73*, no. 224.
9. *CIPM 1347–52*, nos. 297, 590; *CPR 1348–50*, 291.
10. *CIPM 1370–73*, nos. 68, 228–30.
11. *Statutes of the Realm 1100–1377*, 307–09; *CLB F*, 192; *CCR 1349–54*, 87–88.
12. *CPMR*, vol. 1, 225, 229–30.
13. *CPMR*, vol. 1, 226, 228.
14. *CLB F*, 229, and see also the Introduction to this book.
15. *Wills*, vol. 1, 604–05, 635; vol. 2, 86–87, 109; *CLB F*, 222; *CLB G*, 261.
16. *CIPM 1347–52*, no. 483; *CIPM 1352–60*, no. 66; *CCR 1354–60*, 15, 172; *CCR 1399–1402*, 433, 441; *CCR 1405–09*, 4.
17. *CLB F*, 204.
18. *CLB F*, 211; *Wills*, vol. 1, 543–44.
19. *CLB F*, 18, 56, 193–94; *Wills*, vol. 1, 624; *LAN*, nos. 566, 581, 583, 602; *CLB G*, 223, 257, 279, 298–99; CLB H, 13. Walter Burdeyn's father Robert died in 1327: *Wills*, vol. 1, 327–28.

20. *CLB F*, 189; *Memorials of London*, xxxi. William Oyldebeof, or at least someone of this name, was still alive in 1412: *CCR 1409–13*, 321.
21. *CIPM 1336–46*, no. 218; *CIPM 1347–52*, no. 532; *CFR 1327–37*, 115, 124, 317; *CFR 1347–56*, 263, 352–53.

Chapter 21

1. *The Brut or the Chronicles of England*, ed. F.W.D. Brie, part 2, 313–14; The *Anonimalle Chronicle 1333–1381*, ed. V.H. Galbraith, 50; *CLB G*, 138.
2. *CIPM 1377–84*, no. 889.
3. *ODNB*; *Wills*, vol. 2, 61–62.
4. *CIPM 1377–84*, no. 888.
5. *CIPM 1317–27*, no. 662; *CIPM 1370–73*, no. 49; *CIPM 1374–77*, nos. 168, 206.
6. *CIPM 1377–84*, no. 894; www.medievalgenealogy.org.uk/inquests/abstracts_113.shtml, accessed 27 March 2024.
7. *CPR 1358–61*, 337, 571–72, 582–83; *CPR 1361–64*, 1, 6–8; *CIM 1348–77*, no. 460; *CIPM 1352–60*, no. 412; *CCR 1369–74*, 506–07; *CIPM 1370–73*, no. 153.
8. *CCR 1360–64*, 302–03; *CFR 1356–68*, 179, 197, 250; *CIPM 1347–52*, nos. 43, 399; *CIPM 1361–65*, nos. 160–61; *CIPM 1365–69*, no. 177; *CIPM 1399–1405*, nos. 440–45; *CIPM 1418–22*, nos. 453–59.
9. *CIPM 1317–27*, no. 271; *CIPM 1327–36*, nos. 389, 672; *CIPM 1361–65*, nos. 272–73; *CCR 1333–37*, 542, 551; *CFR 1356–68*, 200, 223, 244.
10. *CIPM 1361–65*, no. 187; *CIPM 1374–77*, nos. 81. 298. The Seymour brothers' mother Muriel, born *c.* 1332, was the granddaughter and heir of Richard Lovell of Castle Cary (before 1276–1351).
11. *CIPM 1361–65*, no. 348; *CIPM 1384–92*, nos. 120, 247; *CFR 1356–68*, 230, 246; *CCR 1389–92*, 132–33. An inquisition taken in early 1386 says that Christiana the eldest sister died in July 1364, but Elizabeth's inquisition post mortem of August 1362 gives Isabel alone as her heir, so Christiana must have been dead by then.
12. *CIPM 1307–17*, nos. 464–65; *CIPM 1361–65*, nos. 157–58, 175; *CIPM 1413–18*, nos. 324, 524; *CCR 1318–23*, 306; *CCR 1360–64*, 224.
13. *CIPM 1361–65*, nos. 58, 315; *CIPM 1365–69*, no. 75.
14. *CIPM 1336–46*, nos. 38, 370; *CIPM 1347–52*, no. 594; *CIPM 1361–65*, nos. 34–35; *CIPM 1365–69*, no. 269; *CIPM 1377–84*, nos. 980–81; *CFR 1356–68*, 208; *CCR 1360–64*, 449–50. Alice Beauchamp (d. 1383) was the daughter of Thomas Beauchamp, earl of Warwick (1314–69) and Katherine Mortimer (d. 1369).
15. *CIPM 1336–46*, nos. 148, 655; *CIPM 1361–65*, no. 267; *CIPM 1377–84*, nos. 519–20, 663; *CCR 1360–64*, 251–52; *CCR 1409–13*, 397–98.
16. *CIPM 1361–65*, no. 109.
17. *CIPM 1317–27*, nos. 188, 208, 239; *CIPM 1327–36*, no. 188; *CIPM 1336–46*, no. 443; *CIPM 1361–65*, no. 89; *CIPM 1365–69*, no. 51; *CIPM 1377–84*, no. 665; *CIPM 1413–18*, nos. 787–88; *CCR 1318–23*, 315–16; *CFR 1356–68*, 63, 84, 196, 199, 225; *CCR 1364–68*, 452–53; *CCR 1429–35*, 61.
18. *CIPM 1327–36*, no. 261; *CIPM 1336–46*, no. 33; *CIPM 1347–52*, no. 41; *CIPM 1361–65*, nos. 31–32; *CIPM 1374–77*, no. 118; *CIPM 1392–99*, nos. 335–39; *CIPM 1405–13*, nos. 816–17, 899; *CCR 1346–49*, 325, 367, 460, 506; *CFR 1347–56*, 27, 47; *CCR 1377–81*, 5.
19. *CIPM 1361–65*, no. 119; *CIPM 1374–77*, no. 37; *CIPM 1377–84*, no. 654; *CIPM 1384–92*, no. 704; *CIPM 1405–13*, no. 839.
20. *Wills*, vol. 2, 30, 35; *CLB G*, 228, 320.
21. *Wills*, vol. 2, 31, 34, 44; *CIPM 1370–73*, no. 73.

22. *Wills*, vol. 2, 19–20; *CLB G*, 122, 227.

Chapter 22

1. *CIPM 1327–36*, no. 278; *CIPM 1361–65*, nos. 46, 191.
2. *CIPM 1336–46*, no. 82; *CIPM 1347–52*, no. 52; *CIPM 1361–65*, nos. 195, 432–33.
3. *CIPM 1327–36*, no. 331; *CIPM 1361–65*, no. 427; *CCR 1349–54*, 173.
4. *CIPM 1361–65*, nos. 463–64; *CIPM 1370–73*, no. 291; *CIPM 1374–77*, no. 61; *CFR 1356–68*, 249, 251, 311, 349, 388; *CCR 1374–77*, 29.
5. *CIPM 1347–52*, no. 121; *CIPM 1352–60*, no. 218; *CIPM 1361–65*, no. 87; *CCR 1360–64*, 291–92, 299, 306, 326.
6. *CIPM 1327–36*, no. 558; *CIPM 1361–65*, no. 582; *CIPM 1365–69*, no. 377; *CIPM 1377–84*, no. 974; *CPR 1361–64*, 471; *CCR 1369–74*, 47.
7. www.british-history.ac.uk/vch/hants/vol3/pp94-101; https://thehistoryofparliament.wordpress.com/2020/10/06/the-barbarity-of-the-medieval-criminal-law-petty-treason-and-the-murders-of-sir-thomas-murdak-and-john-cotell/, both accessed 10 March 2024.
8. *CIPM 1361–65*, no. 368; *CIPM 1377–84*, no. 452; *CCR 1381–85*, 5.
9. *CIPM 1352–60*, no. 90; *CIPM 1365–59*, no. 407.
10. *CIPM 1327–36*, no. 68; *CIPM 1347–52*, no. 426; *CIPM 1361–65*, nos. 90, 93; *CIPM 1365–69*, no. 228. John and Christine's son John had a son also called John born around Christmas 1362, and died in 1368.
11. *CIPM 1336–46*, no. 26; *CIPM 1361–65*, no. 56; *CIPM 1399–1405*, no. 1000; *CPR 1334–38*, 345.
12. *CIPM 1361–65*, nos. 244, 313; *CIPM 1365–69*, no. 135; *CIPM 1370–73*, no. 11; *CIPM 1377–84*, nos. 462–63.
13. *CIPM 1361–65*, nos. 243, 246; *CCR 1360–64*, 319.
14. *CIPM 1361–65*, no. 83; *CIPM 1365–69*, no. 375; CIPM 1412–18, nos. 211–17; *CCR 1360–64*, 304.
15. *CIPM 1347–52*, no. 233; *CIPM 1361–65*, nos. 107, 230, 253–54; *CCR 1360–64*, 237, 372.
16. *Wills*, vol. 2, 63; *CLB G*, 156; *CLB H*, 305.
17. *Wills*, vol. 2, 47; CIPM 1317–27, nos. 181–82, 632; *CIPM 1352–60*, nos. 623 24; *CIPM 1361–65*, nos. 147–49, 252; *CIPM 1413–18*, no. 157; *CCR 1360–64*, 303–04, 339, 512, 514–15.
18. *CIPM 1361–65*, nos. 152–53, 541; *CIPM 1365–69*, no. 400; *CIPM 1384–92*, nos.479–80, 882; *CIPM 1405–13*, no. 402; *CIPM 1422–27*, no. 660.
19. *CIPM 1327–36*, no. 535; *CIPM 1361–65*, no. 71; *CIPM 1374–77*, no. 157; *CIPM 1399–1405*, no. 979; *CCR 1333–37*, 66–67; *CPR 1377–81*, 64.
20. *CIPM 1361–65*, nos. 398–99.
21. *CIPM 1361–65*, nos. 178–79; *CIPM 1374–77*, no. 53; *CIPM 1405–13*, no. 64.
22. *Wills*, vol. 2, 59–60; *CLB H*, 445.
23. *CIPM 1352–60*, no. 653; *CIPM 1361–65*, nos. 1, 222; *CIPM 1365–69*, no. 387.
24. *Wills*, vol. 2, 48; *CLB G*, 157, 332; *CLB H*, 14, 17.
25. *Wills*, vol. 2, 60–61; *CLB G*, 134–35, 155, 235.
26. *CIPM 1352–60*, nos. 141, 190; *CIPM 1361–65*, no. 138; *Wills*, vol. 2, 38; *CLB G*, 207; *CCR 1369–74*, 155. John Malweyn the elder had outlived his wife Margery, one of the two daughters and co-heirs of Augustine and Maud Waleys. John Dovy married a woman called Katherine instead: *CCR 1364–68*, 491; *CCR 1369–74*, 291, 343, and see also Chapter 24.
27. *CIPM 1361–65*, no. 33; *CFR 1356–68*, 187, 200; *CCR 1402–05*, 172.
28. *CIPM 1361–65*, no. 200.

29. *CIPM 1361–65*, 136, 594; *CIPM 1399–1405*, no. 876; *CIPM 1405–13*, no. 360; *CIPM 1413–18*, no. 283; *CFR 1356–68*, 174, 190, 198, 291, 300.
30. *Wills*, vol. 1, 276, 544; vol. 2, 57–58; *CLB D*, 47, 49, 161; *CLB G*, 256–57.

Chapter 23

1. *Brut or the Chronicles of England*, part 2, 321.
2. *Wills*, vol. 2, 125.
3. *CIM 1348–77*, no. 698.
4. *CIPM 1374–77*, no. 344.
5. *CIPM 1352–60*, no. 497; *CIPM 1361–65*, no. 508; *CIPM 1365–69*, nos. 377, 380; *CIPM 1377–84*, no. 51.
6. *CIPM 1327–36*, nos. 18, 317; *CIPM 1336–46*, no. 53; *CIPM 1347–52*, no. 225; *CIPM 1365–69*, no. 381; *CIPM 1392–99*, no. 1174; 1399–1405, nos. 232–33.
7. *Testamenta Vetusta*, vol. 1, 78–80; *CIPM 1307–17*, no. 615; *CIPM 1365–69*, no. 326. *The Complete Peerage*, vol. 12B, 374, says he died of plague, though does not cite a source.
8. *Wills*, vol. 2, 117–18.
9. *Wills*, vol. 2, 114; *CPMR*, vol. 3, 28 note 50; *CCR 1360–64*, 239.
10. *CIPM 1336–46*, nos. 338, 505; *CIPM 1352–60*, no. 105; *CFR 1337–47*, 367; *CFR 1347–56*, 374, 393–94; *CPR 1338–40*, 440–41; *CCR 1364–68*, 107–08.
11. *CIPM 1365–69*, nos. 242, 402, 406; *CIPM 1377–84*, no. 656; *Testamenta Eboracensia, Or, Wills Registered at York*, vol. 1, ed. James Raine, 201–02 (*meum primerium viride quod quondam fuit domini patris mei*).
12. *CIPM 1365–69*, no. 415; *CIPM 1374–77*, no. 201.
13. *Wills*, vol. 1, 598; *Wills*, vol. 2, 127–28; *CLB G*, 7, 12; *A Descriptive Catalogue of Ancient Deeds*, vol. 2, no. C4216.
14. *CIPM 1361–65*, nos. 116–17; *CIPM 1374–77*, nos. 40, 41, 67; *CCR 1374–77*, 54–56, 134.
15. *CIPM 1352–60*, no. 546; *CIPM 1365–69*, nos. 369, 439, 441.
16. *CIPM 1365–69*, no. 408; *CIPM 1370–73*, no. 47; *CIPM 1374–77*, no. 52; *CFR 1369–77*, 77, 119, 129; *CCR 1369–74*, 142, 144, 322; *CPR 1367–70*, 472; *CCR 1374–77*, 450; *CCR 1377–81*, 67–68.
17. *CIPM 1291–1300*, no. 227; *CIPM 1317–27*, no. 279; *CIPM 1336–46*, no. 443; *CIPM 1347–52*, no. 189; *CIPM 1365–69*, nos. 170, 417; *CIPM 1432–37*, nos. 318–19, 457.
18. *Wills*, vol. 2, 118–19, 261, 267, 378–79; *CLB G*, 234; *CLB I*, 127.
19. *CIPM 1365–69*, no. 404; *CIPM 1370–73*, no. 69.
20. *CIPM 1327–36*, nos. 150, 179; *CIPM 1365–69*, nos. 364, 392–93; *CIPM 1392–99*, no. 98; *CFR 1369–77*, 53, 56–57.

Chapter 24

1. *Anonimalle Chronicle*, 77, 79; Brut, part 2, 328; *John of Gaunt's Register*, Part 1, 1371–1375, vol. 2, ed. Sydney Armitage-Smith, no. 1696, *le peril que pourroit avenir de ceste pestilence q'ore est.*
2. *CIPM 1347–52*, no. 428; *CIPM 1361–65*, no. 442; *CIPM 1365–69*, no. 421; *CIPM 1370–73*, no. 128; *CIPM 1374–77*, no. 212.
3. *CIPM 1361–65*, no. 345; *CIPM 1374–77*, no. 161; *CIPM 1392–99*, no. 276; *CCR 1374–77*, 163.
4. *CIPM 1374–77*, no. 111.
5. *CIPM 1327–36*, no. 288; *CIPM 1347–52*, no. 16; *CIPM 1370–73*, no. 241; *CIPM 1374–77*, nos. 152–54; *CIPM 1399–1405*, nos. 400–03; *CIPM 1418–22*, nos. 797–99;

CIPM 1422–27, no. 515; *CFR 1369–77*, 202, 207, 293, 319, 324–25; *CCR 1374–77*, 156, 183–84, 193–94, 318–19, 359.

6. *Wills*, vol. 2, 174, 388–89; *CCR 1374–77*, 259, 266; *CIPM 1399–1405*, no. 625.
7. *Wills*, vol. 2, 124, 169–70, 201, 253.
8. *Wills*, vol. 2, 153–54, 178, 527; *CPMR*, vol. 2, 207.
9. *Wills*, vol. 2, 176–77.
10. *CIPM 1374–77*, nos. 191–92.
11. *CIPM 1370–73*, no. 273; *CIPM 1374–77*, nos. 197, 237; *CIPM 1418–22*, nos. 189–91.
12. *CIPM 1370–73*, no. 278; *CIPM 1374–77*, no. 203. Agnes's uncle Geoffrey was the godson of Sir Geoffrey Luttrell (1276–1345) of the Luttrell Psalter: *Early Lincoln Wills: An Abstract of All the Wills and Administrations Recorded in the Episcopal Registers of the Old Diocese of Lincoln*, 1280–1547, ed. Alfred Gibbons (1888), 18.
13. *CIPM 1370–73*, no. 106; *CIPM 1374–77*, no. 142; *CIPM 1377–84*, no. 231; *CFR 1369–77*, 326; *CCR 1374–77*, 434–35; *CCR 1377–81*, 63–64.
14. *CIPM 1374–77*, no. 188; *CIPM 1384–92*, no. 924.
15. *Abstracts of Inquisitiones Post Mortem for Gloucestershire*, vol. 5, 1302–1358, ed. Edward Alexander Fry, 285–86, 314–15, 368–69; *CIPM 1336–46*, no. 325; *CIPM 1347–52*, no. 13; *CIPM 1352–60*, no. 449; *CIPM 1374–77*, no. 143; *CIPM 1413–18*, no. 684.
16. *CIPM 1374–77*, no. 338; *CIPM 1392–99*, no. 883; *CIPM 1399–2405*, no. 6; *CCR 1389–92*, 146; *CCR 1392–96*, 474.
17. *CIPM 1365–69*, no. 312; *CIPM 1374–77*, no. 323; *CFR 1369–77*, 56; *CCR 1369–74*, 91, 93, 122; *CPR 1364–67*, 126; *CPR 1370–74*, 115; *CPR 1389–92*, 246; *CPR 1408–13*, 350–51, 358.
18. *Wills*, vol. 2, 9, 181, 235; *CLB H*, 82; Court of Common Pleas, CP 40/655, rot. 111, available on British History Online.
19. *Wills*, vol. 1, 545, 699; vol. 2, 184.
20. *Wills*, vol. 2, 179–80; *CLB H*, 15.
21. *Wills*, vol. 1, 672–73; *Wills*, vol. 2, 166; *CIPM 1374–77*, no. 2; *CLB H*, 8–9.
22. *Wills*, vol. 2, 162–63.
23. *CIPM 1347–52*, no. 653; *CIPM 1374–77*, no. 97; *CIPM 1392–99*, nos. 142–43; *CIPM 1422–27*, no. 750; *CIPM 1432–27*, nos. 604–06; *CCR 1374–77*, 163–64; *CCR 1389–92*, 271–72. In 1362, John Lokton's father Thomas Lokton took part in the proof of age of Alice Cornwalays, whose father Robert died on 14 August 1349 (see Chapter 18), and said that his daughter Katherine died in the month Alice was born, August 1337: *CIPM 1361–65*, no. 382.
24. *CIPM 1374–77*, nos. 127, 216, 290; *CFR 1369–77*, 323, 349; *CCR 1374–77*, 315–16.
25. *CIPM 1374–77*, nos. 222, 291; *CIPM 1377–84*, no. 64; *CIPM 1384–92*, no. 1046; *CCR 1392–96*, 60.
26. *CIPM 1336–46*, no. 457; *CIPM 1352–60*, no. 529; *CIPM 1365–69*, no. 126; *CIPM 1370–73*, nos. 141, 219; *CIPM 1374–77*, nos. 22, 124–25; *CIPM 1405–13*, nos. 34–38; *CIPM 1413–18*, no. 267; *CIPM 1427–32*, nos. 212–13, 665; *CCR 1343–46*, 35; TNA E 40/12138.
27. *Wills*, vol. 2, 119–20, 185, 191–92; *CLB G*, 286; *CLB H*, 44, 103, 141; *CPMR*, vol. 2, 223; *LAN*, no. 586.
28. *Wills*, vol. 2, 185–86; *CLB H*, 3–4, 31–32, 35.

Afterwards

1. *The Westminster Chronicle 1381–1394*, ed. and trans. L.C. Hector and B.F. Harvey (1982), 440–41.

Bibliography

Primary Sources

Abstracts of Coroners' Inquests in Northamptonshire, www.medievalgenealogy.org.uk/inquests/index.shtml

Abstracts of Feet of Fines, www.medievalgenealogy.org.uk/fines/search.php

An Abstract for the Feet of Fines for the County of Sussex, vol. 3, ed. L.F. Salzmann (1916)

Abstracts of Feet of Fines for Wiltshire for the Reign of Edward III, ed. C.R. Elrington (1974)

Abstracts of Inquisitiones Post Mortem for Gloucestershire, vol. 5, 1302–1358, ed. Edward Alexander Fry, and vol. 6, 1359–1413, ed. Ethel Stokes (1910–14)

The Anonimalle Chronicle 1333–1381, ed. V.H. Galbraith (second edition, 1970)

The Black Death, ed. and trans. Rosemary Horrox (1994)

British History Online, www.british-history.ac.uk/

The Brut or the Chronicles of England, part 2, ed. F.W.D. Brie (1908)

Calendar of Close Rolls, thirty-one vols., 1307–1435 (1892–1933)

Calendar of Coroners Rolls of the City of London 1300–1378, ed. Reginald R. Sharpe (1913)

Calendar of Entries in the Papal Registers Relating to Great Britain and Ireland: Papal Letters, vol. 3, 1342–62, ed. W.H. Bliss and C. Johnson (1897)

Calendar of Fine Rolls, twelve vols., 1272–1405 (1911–31)

Calendar of Inquisitions Miscellaneous, vol. 2, 1308–48, and vol. 3, 1348–77 (1916–37)

Calendar of Inquisitions Post Mortem, twenty-four vols., 1291–1447 (1912–2009)

Calendar of Letter-Books of the City of London, Letter-Book E (1314–37), *Letter-Book F* (1337–52), *Letter-Book G* (1352–74) and *Letter-Book H* (1375–99), ed. Reginald R. Sharpe (1903–07)

Calendar of Patent Rolls, thirty-one vols., 1301–1408 (1898–1907)

Calendar of the Plea and Memoranda Rolls of the City of London, vol. 1, 1323–64, vol. 2, 1364–81, and vol. 3, 1381–1412, ed. A.H. Thomas (1926–32)

Calendar of Wills Proved and Enrolled in the Court of Husting, London, vol. 1, 1258–1358, and vol. 2, 1358–1688, ed. Reginald R. Sharpe (1889–90)

Chronicon Galfridi le Baker de Swynbroke, ed. E.M. Thompson (1899)

A Descriptive Catalogue of Ancient Deeds, six vols., ed. H.C. Maxwell Lyte (1890–1915)

Early Lincoln Wills: An Abstract of All the Wills and Administrations Recorded in the Episcopal Registers of the Old Diocese of Lincoln, 1280–1547, ed. Alfred Gibbons (1888)

Feet of Fines for the County of Somerset 1347–1399, ed. Emanuel Green (1902)

Feet of Fines for Essex, vol. 2, ed. Ernest F. Kirk (1913)

Foedera, Conventiones, Litterae et Cujuscunque Generis Acta Publica, vol. 3, part 1, 1344–61, ed. Thomas Rymer (1825)

Inquisitions and Assessments Relating to Feudal Aids 1284–1431, 6 vols. (1899–1920)

John of Gaunt's Register, Part 1, 1371–75, two vols., ed. Sydney Armitage-Smith (1911)

Life Records of Chaucer, Parts 1 to 4, ed. Walford D. Selby, F.J. Furnivall, Edward A. Bond and R.E.G. Kirk (1900)

London Assize of Nuisance, 1301–1431: A Calendar, ed. Helena M. Chew and William Kellaway (1973)
*Memorials of London and London Life in the 13*th, *14*th *and 15*th *Centuries*, ed. H.T. Riley (1868)
The Parliament Rolls of Medieval England, ed. Chris Given-Wilson, Paul Brand, Seymour Phillips, Mark Ormrod, Geoffrey Martin, Anne Curry and Rosemary Horrox (2005)
Petitions to the Pope 1342–1419, ed. W.H. Bliss (1896)
Polychronicon Ranulphi Higden Monachi Cestrensis, vol. 8, ed. Joseph Rawson Lumby (1882)
Records of the Borough of Leicester, vol. 2, 1326–1509, ed. Mary Bateson (1901)
Register of Edward, the Black Prince, vol. 4, ed. M.C.B. Dawes (1933)
Staffordshire Historical Collections, vol. 7, part 1, ed. George Wrottesley (1886)
Staffordshire Historical Collections, vol. 11, ed. George Wrottesley and F. Parker (1890)
Statutes of the Realm, vol. 1, 1101–1377 (1810)
Testamenta Eboracensia, Or, Wills Registered at York, vol. 1, ed. James Raine (1836)
Testamenta Vetusta: Being Illustrations from Wills, vol. 1, ed. Nicholas Harris Nicolas (1826)
The Westminster Chronicle 1381–1394, ed. and trans. L.C. Hector and B.F. Harvey (1982)

Selected Secondary Sources

A History of the County of Wiltshire, vol. 4 (1959), available on British History Online
Beltz, George Frederick, *Memorials of the Order of the Garter* (1841)
Bennett, Judith M. and Shannon McSheffrey, 'Early, Erotic and Alien: Women Dressed as Men in Late Medieval London', *History Workshop Journal*, 77 (2014), 1–25
Bennett, Nicholas Hamilton, 'The Beneficed Clergy in the Diocese of Lincoln during the Episcopate of Henry Burghersh, 1320–1340', Univ. of York DPhil thesis (1989)
Bullock-Davies, Constance, *Menestrellorum Multitudo: Minstrels at a Royal Feast* (1978)
The Complete Peerage of England, Scotland, Ireland, Great Britain and the United Kingdom, vol. 7, ed. G.E.C. (1896)
Gummer, Benedict, *The Scourging Angel: The Black Death in the British Isles* (2009)
The History of Parliament Online https://www.historyofparliamentonline.org/
Keene, D.J., and Vanessa Harding, *Historical Gazetteer of London Before the Great Fire Cheapside; Parishes of All Hallows Honey Lane, St Martin Pomary, St Mary Le Bow, St Mary Colechurch and St Pancras Soper Lane* (1987)
Kelly, John, *The Great Mortality: An Intimate History of the Black Death* (2005)
Megson, Barbara E., 'Mortality Among London Citizens in the Black Death', *Medieval Prosopography*, 19 (1998), 125–33
Newton, Stella Mary, *Fashion in the Age of the Black Prince* (1980)
Ormrod, W.M., 'The Royal Nursery: A Household for the Younger Children of Edward III', *English Historical Review*, 120 (2005), 398–415
Ormrod, W. Mark, *Edward III* (2011)
Oxford Dictionary of National Biography, online edition
Redstone, Vincent B. and Lilian J., 'The Heyrons of London: A Study in the Social Origins of Geoffrey Chaucer', *Speculum*, 12 (1937), 182–95
Sloane, Barney, *The Black Death in London* (2011)
Stern, Derek Vincent, *A Hertfordshire Demesne of Westminster Abbey* (2000)
Watney, John, *Some Account of the Hospital of St Thomas of Acon, in the Cheap, London, and of the Plate of the Mercers' Company* (1892)
Woolgar, C.M., *The Great Household in Late Medieval England* (1999)

Index